Deep Tissue Massage

Hands-On Guides for Therapists

Deep Tissue Massage

Hands-On Guides for Therapists

Jane Johnson, MCSP, MSc

Human Kinetics

Library of Congress Cataloging-in-Publication Data

Johnson, Jane, 1965-
  Deep tissue massage / Jane Johnson.
     p. ; cm. -- (Hands-on guides for therapists)
  Includes bibliographical references and index.
  ISBN-13: 978-0-7360-8470-3 (soft cover)
  ISBN-10: 0-7360-8470-3 (soft cover)
  1. Massage therapy. I. Title. II. Series: Hands-on guides for therapists.
  [DNLM: 1. Massage--methods. WB 537 J67d 2011]
  RM721.J644 2011
  615.8'2--dc22
                                    2010006740

ISBN: 978-0-7360-8470-3 (print)

Acquisitions Editor: John Dickinson, PhD; **Developmental Editor:** Amanda S. Ewing; **Assistant Editor:** Casey A. Gentis; **Copyeditor:** John Wentworth; **Permission Manager:** Dalene Reeder; **Graphic Designer:** Nancy Rasmus; **Graphic Artist:** Angela K. Snyder; **Cover Designer:** Keith Blomberg; **Photographer (cover):** Neil Bernstein; **Photographer (interior):** Neil Bernstein; **Visual Production Assistant:** Joyce Brumfield; **Photo Production Manager:** Jason Allen; **Art Manager:** Kelly Hendren; **Associate Art Manager:** Alan L. Wilborn; **Illustrators:** Jason M. McAlexander, MFA, and Alan L. Wilborn; **Printer:** McNaughton & Gunn

Special thanks to Douglas Nelson, LMT, for his expertise as the massage therapist in the photographs.

Printed in the United States of America   10   9   8   7

The paper in this book is certified under a sustainable forestry program.

Human Kinetics
1607 N. Market Street
Champaign, IL 61820
USA

United States and International
Website: **US.HumanKinetics.com**
Email: info@hkusa.com
Phone: 1-800-747-4457

Canada
Website: **Canada.HumanKinetics.com**
Email: info@hkcanada.com

E4898

Tell us what you think!
Human Kinetics would love to hear what we can do to improve the customer experience. Use this QR code to take our brief survey.

Contents

PART III Applying Deep Tissue Massage

PART IV   Deep Tissue Massage Routines and Programmes

Massage may be one of the oldest therapies still used today. At present more therapists than ever before are practicing an ever-expanding range of massage techniques. Many of these techniques are taught through massage schools and within degree courses. Our need now is to provide the best clinical and educational resources that will enable massage therapists to learn the required techniques for delivering massage therapy to clients. Human Kinetics has developed the Hands-On Guides for Therapists series with this in mind.

The Hands-On Guides for Therapists series provides specific tools of assessment and treatment that fall well within the realm of massage therapists but may also be useful for other bodyworkers, such as osteopaths and fitness instructors. Each book in the series is a step-by-step guide to delivering the techniques to clients. Each book features a full-colour interior packed with photos illustrating every technique. Tips provide handy advice to help you adjust your technique, and the Client Talk boxes contain examples of how the techniques can be used with clients who have particular problems. Throughout each book are questions that enable you to test your knowledge and skill, which will be particularly helpful if you are attempting to pass a qualification exam. We've even provided the answers too!

You might be using a book from the Hands-On Guides for Therapists series to obtain the required skills to help you pass a course or to brush up on skills you learned in the past. You might be a course tutor looking for ways to make massage therapy come alive with your students. This series provides easy-to-follow steps that will make the transition from theory to practice seem effortless. The Hands-On Guides for Therapists series is an essential resource for all those who are serious about massage therapy.

Preface

Many clients enjoy the sensation of deep tissue massage, and when asked for their preferences beforehand, these clients request 'firm' or 'deep' pressure. Yet some therapists shy away from incorporating this form of massage into their treatments, believing it to require the application of force greater than that of which they can deliver. Therapists also may be anxious about how to apply pressure safely. This book was written for those of you searching for ways to increase the depth of pressure you use in a manner that is both safe and effective for yourself and your clients. Here you will find simple explanations of how to use compressive and stretching techniques while applying them in ways that facilitate additional leverage to tissues. By following the guidelines provided, along with a little practice, this book will help you to deliver massage in such a way that your clients perceive a comfortable and considerable increase in the pressure they receive from your treatments.

You will also find the book useful if you are an experienced therapist looking for techniques to avoid overuse of your hands. Ideas are presented for the use of forearms, fists and elbows. Or perhaps you are already skilled in the use of deep tissue massage and are looking to add variety to your existing treatments. If you are a teacher of massage, you may find ideas and alternatives to stimulate debate within the classroom. Whatever your aims, in this book you will find plentiful photographs, tips and tricks to inform and inspire.

To get you started, Part I introduces this form of massage, its effects and benefits. This part also covers important safety issues and provides clear guidelines for the correct use of your own body and for the use of massage tools. Part II describes two main methods for applying deep tissue massage—compressive techniques (chapter 3) and stretching techniques (chapter 4).

In part III, the chapters are organized by body part. Chapter 5 contains deep tissue massage techniques for the muscles of the trunk while chapter 6 covers the lower limbs. Last in this part, chapter 7 covers the upper limbs. In each of these chapters you will find techniques for the application of deep tissue massage provided for prone, supine and three-quarter lying positions.

Finally, part IV concentrates on deep tissue massage routines. Use this part of the book to help you practice using the techniques in one particular position before moving on to the next position.

Whether you are a newly qualified therapist or a therapist with many years of experience, I encourage you to experiment with this material by giving and receiving the techniques described here. Discover those techniques and treatment positions that appeal to you and discard those which you find less helpful. With practice, you will find many of these techniques easy to apply and will quickly be able to include them as part of your routine. As always, it is my intention to help disseminate information regarding the practice of massage. Please share these techniques with other therapists and as always, feel free to get in touch with me with your comments and suggestions regarding the material presented.

Acknowledgments

I would like to start by thanking massage therapist Douglas Nelson, LMT, who has once again managed to reproduce treatment positions and hand holds based on my original photographs; this time for deep tissue massage techniques. Thank you also to Abraham Jones and Rebecca Ray for modelling for us.

I commend developmental editor Amanda Ewing for making so few changes to my manuscript, John Wentworth for his copyediting, and Nancy Rasmus for the uncomplicated design of this series, *Hands-On Guides for Therapists*.

I would also like to acknowledge the invaluable input I derived from all of the therapists who have, over the years, attended my workshops on deep tissue massage. I hope this book goes some way in answering your questions.

Finally, I would like to thank John Dickinson, acquisitions editor at Human Kinetics, for offering me the opportunity to write this book in the first place.

PART I

Getting Started With Deep Tissue Massage Techniques

Congratulations on wanting to learn more about deep tissue massage. In chapter 1 you will be introduced to the main methods for achieving deep tissue massage and the effects that these compressive and stretching techniques have on the body. You will also discover the benefits of this kind of treatment for both you and your clients, and how this type of massage differs from sports massage. Also included is advice on where and when deep tissue massage should be performed and some general tips on how to increase the depth of your massage (an area that we revisit in more detail in part II, where you will really get to grips with the different methods of application).

Chapter 2 covers everything you need to help you prepare to give a deep tissue massage. We help you identify your treatment goals and explore the concept of working with intent. The section on safety guidelines helps to ensure that you work safely and effectively with these deep tissue techniques. The chapter's troubleshooting tips and answers to frequently asked questions address many common queries and concerns. In these two chapters of part I and throughout the book you will find quick questions at the end of each chapter. Use these questions to test yourself and to reinforce what you have read. Answers to the quick questions appear at the end of the book.

Introduction to Deep Tissue Massage

In this first chapter we will set the scene for deep tissue massage by exploring the concepts involved in its application. The two main methods of application are to compress tissues and to stretch tissues. Understanding the effects of these techniques (individually and combined) will help you make informed judgements about which of your clients might benefit most from deep tissue massage. This chapter also helps prepare you for chapters 3 and 4, in which the application of these techniques is covered in detail.

Also presented in this chapter are answers to commonly asked questions: How do you increase the depth of your massage? How is deep tissue massage different from sports massage? What are the effects and benefits of deep tissue massage? Last but not least, we'll examine where and when deep tissue massage can be performed.

What Are the Methods of Application?

Manual massage consists of five well-known techniques: effleurage, petrissage, tapotement, frictions and vibrations, each of which can be performed in a variety of ways. These are the strokes that form the basis of Swedish massage, and their effects vary according to factors such as the strength and speed with which they are delivered and the physical and emotional states of both the recipient and the therapist providing them. In this book you are going to learn how compressive and stretching techniques can be used to help you work more deeply into tissues—the skin, muscles and their supportive fascia—if this is your intention. There are many variants on how these techniques can be applied, which together form the basis of deep tissue massage.

Compressive Techniques

You are already using compressive techniques: broadly and lightly when you effleurage, more firmly and with a wringing motion when you petrissage, and during 'holding' techniques whenever you hold a muscle or lift it away from underlying structures. You might even be using your fingers or thumbs to apply deep localized digital pressure to specific spots on a muscle, such as when treating trigger spots. Here you are going to learn how to apply deep pressure while safeguarding your hands, fingers and thumbs, and in doing so you will explore the best ways to use your forearms, fists and elbows. Squeezing techniques are also discussed, as is advice on the use of massage tools, which is valuable for compressing specific spots on a muscle. You will learn how to apply each of these compressive techniques statically, and then how they can be combined with stretching techniques to provide really deep tissue massage.

Tapotement is a form of compression but will not be discussed here. The short, sudden strike of these percussive techniques (e.g., hacking, clapping and beating) compress tissues suddenly and rapidly and are stimulatory in nature, aimed at inducing vasodilation, vibrating tissues and triggering cutaneous reflexes. The compressive techniques described in this book are slow, sustained and aimed at facilitating deep relaxation and a reduction, rather than an increase, in the tone of muscles. Everything you need to know about the application of compressive techniques you will find in chapter 3.

To start, see figure 1.1 a-e; these illustrations show the effect of different types of compression. The layered-looking boxes represent a cross section of skin, muscle and bone. Fascia is not shown but is found beneath the skin and wraps around and invaginates muscles, as you know.

You may have heard the riddle: 'Which makes the deeper impression into a carpet—an elephant's footprint or a lady's stiletto-heeled shoe?' Many people quickly answer the footprint of the elephant because the elephant is so heavy. However, when applied to the same kind of surface and using the same weight, penetration is deeper when applied to a smaller surface area. So the lady's heel may well leave the deeper impression on the carpet, although she is obviously much lighter than an elephant. Her heel directs weight to a small, localized area, whereas the broad flat pad of the elephant's foot disperses weight over a larger surface area, thus making a less deep impression in the carpet. Understanding this helps us when working with the compressive techniques needed for deep tissue massage.

Notice that the depth of compression achieved using a massage tool (1.1e) is equal to the depth of compression when using your elbow (1.1d), although the tool covers a smaller surface area. The reason is that you are usually at a slight mechanical disadvantage when using a massage tool and thus not able to deliver as much weight. This is also the case when using your fist. The fist covers a smaller surface area (1.1c), so you would expect to be able to press more deeply into tissues than when using your forearm (1.1b). However, when using your fist or a massage tool, you often work with your arms held straight, directing pressure through your elbows and wrists, which need to be kept in a neutral position. Maintaining this position with your arms requires more effort than when using your forearms (in which case you simply lean on the client, transferring your body weight to him or her).

Notice too just how deeply you can compress tissues when using your elbow or a massage tool. You could press the tissues right up to and onto the underlying bone, but this is neither safe nor desirable. Remember this when working on thinner muscles and those that lie close to the bone.

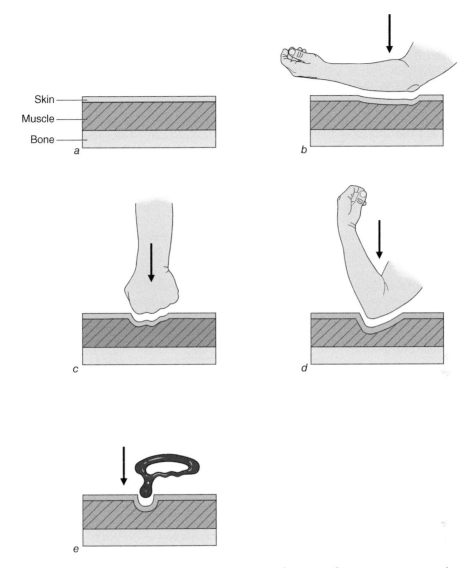

Figure 1.1 Types of compression: *(a)* noncompressed tissues, *(b)* tissues compressed using the forearm, *(c)* tissues compressed using the fist, *(d)* tissues compressed using the elbow and *(e)* tissues compressed using a massage tool.

Understand that the illustrations in figure 1.1 are designed to help you differentiate the effects of different forms of compression. How much you actually compress tissues will depend on your strength and leverage, as well as on which sort of tissues you are compressing and the state of those tissues. Muscles depress more readily than tendons; muscles with a high state of tone are harder to compress than those with a lower state of tone. Clients with muscle tension are more likely to sense your pressure as being 'deep' compared to when the same pressure is applied to clients whose muscles are relaxed. So, although you will learn how to compress tissue very deeply, you will not always want to do so.

Stretching Techniques

Whenever you massage, you stretch tissues. Unless you are using very large amounts of oil and a feather-like touch, even light effleurage stretches the skin slightly. In this book you're going to learn how the stretching of skin, fascia and muscles can be specifically incorporated into your massage treatment. Unlike the kind of stretching you might perform after exercise, or a passive stretch you might incorporate at the end of a treatment for your client, the kinds of stretching described here are specific to the application of deep tissue massage. You will learn a variety of stretching techniques both with and without the use of oil, plus how to enhance these with tractioning of a limb. Moving the joint associated with the muscles on which you are working can also be used to increase stretch in tissues, and this technique is also presented. Together, these stretching techniques are intended for use as part of a massage treatment, and you will find many tips and tricks on how to apply them safely and effectively in chapter 4. You will also learn where they are best used on the body.

Figure 1.2 presents more diagrams that might help you visualize the effects of stretch on skin and muscles (figures 1.2a and b). As you can see in figure 1.2a, with lots of oil and little compression you glide across the skin, and there is very little stretch. The effect here would not be considered deep tissue massage. However, with no (or less) oil (figure 1.2b), you may grip the skin and stretch it, and this shearing force might stretch the underlying fascia and muscle too slightly.

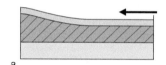 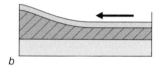

a   b

Figure 1.2   Stretch on skin and muscle: (a) effect of stretch when lots of oil is used, and (b) effect of stretch when little or no oil is used.

Combining Compression and Stretch Techniques

Finally, notice what happens when you combine the forces of compression and stretch (figure 1.3). When compression and stretch are used together, the therapist usually angles the direction of pressure so that it is no longer perpendicular to the tissues but instead acts on them obliquely. The result is that while the tissues are physically compressed less deeply, clients often report *feeling* a deep compression. This might be because the stretch receptors in the client's muscles and tendons are activated, signaling stretching sensations to the brain.

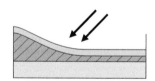

Figure 1.3   Effect of compression and stretch.

Modifications and combinations of the forces of compression and stretch provide you with a wide variety of treatment options. For example, using oil and a broad surface area (such as the forearm) provides lighter compression and little stretch; using less oil and a smaller surface area (such as the elbow) provides deep compression and greater stretch.

How Do You Increase the Depth of Your Massage?

Whether you are a newly qualified massage therapist or have been working as a therapist for many years, you have likely come across clients who enjoy the sensation of deep tissue massage. Mechanically, there are five things you can do to increase the depth of your massage. Let's look briefly at each of the five.

1. Apply more pressure. Many therapists discount this possibility, believing they are not physically capable of applying more pressure, perhaps because they are tiny compared to their client, or because their client is particularly muscular. Lacking confidence, therapists sometimes avoid treating clients who request deep tissue massage, doubting their ability to compress tissues any more than they are already doing. As you will learn in chapter 2, there are ways to use your body and equipment to dramatically increase pressure irrespective of your body weight.

CLIENT TALK

Many years ago I was asked to provide a workshop on deep tissue massage to a group of Japanese aromatherapists. The group was comprised of female therapists, most of them slight of frame. The therapists were initially dubious that they would be able to use deep tissue techniques, but after lowering all the treatment couches and practicing on each other, they discovered that with proper leverage and by using the right technique they could apply deep tissue massage quite effectively.

2. Keep the pressure the same, but reduce the surface area to which you are applying it. In chapter 3, you will explore what happens when you reduce the surface area for compression, comparing the different effects of using your forearm, fist, elbow or a massage tool.
3. Apply more pressure *and* reduce the surface area to which you are applying pressure.
4. Have the client contract the muscle that works opposite to the one you are treating (i.e., the antagonist muscle). Contraction of the antagonist results in a decrease in tone in the agonist (the muscle you are working), thus facilitating deeper pressure. Some of the techniques we will describe in this book make use of this characteristic of muscle function.
5. Give the impression of deep pressure without physically pressing into tissue more deeply. Here we come to one of the tricks of the trade of deep tissue massage. The sensation of deep pressure occurs when you add a stretching component to your massage. Everything you need to know about this is covered in chapter 4, in which you will explore how to stretch tissues with and without oil, combining them with compression for maximum effect.

How Is Deep Tissue Massage Different From Sports Massage?

Sports massage may include the five basic massage strokes combined with more advanced techniques, used to address specific problems such as muscle cramp, excessively tight muscles, joint stiffness or excessive scar tissue. Sports massage might also be used to help athletes prepare for sporting events and to aid recovery following exercise. Sports massage might include specialist techniques such as soft tissue release (STR), muscle energy technique (MET) or proprioceptive neuromuscular facilitation (PNF) used in isolation or combined with other aspects of the overall treatment. Deep tissue massage is simply another skill that is quite useful to the sports massage therapist.

How deep tissue massage is applied when used as part of a sports massage treatment will vary: different mediums (e.g., oil, wax, balm, cream) are used, and therapists use their own combinations of compression and stretch to facilitate the desired treatment outcome. Deep tissue massage *can* be used as a stand-alone treatment by any massage therapist, but it is unlikely that clients would want or need their entire treatment to consist of deep tissue massage. More commonly, deep tissue techniques are used when therapists need to access a muscle more deeply (e.g., to facilitate lengthening of the muscle or to promote an increase in range in the associated joint) or when clients particularly like the sensation of deep massage on parts of their body. Many therapists who are not sports massage therapists find deep tissue massage techniques well worth learning because the techniques enable them to treat a wider variety of clients and conditions.

What Are the Effects of Deep Tissue Massage?

Let's now look at what can happen from a physiological point of view when we compress and stretch tissues. Some effects might be readily apparent, such as an increase in joint range. Other effects might be more subtle and less observable, such as a functional realignment of muscle fibers.

Effects of Compression

Whatever method you choose to compress tissues (with forearm, fist, elbow or a massage tool, or by gripping a muscle and squeezing it), through compression you temporarily impede blood flow to an area by squashing off the stream of blood to small vessels. Once pressure is reduced, these vessels are no longer compressed and fresh blood floods the area.

Imagine a garden lawn strewn with water hoses. The lawn represents the muscles of the body, and the hoses represent the arterioles and capillaries serving the muscles by providing the oxygen and nutrients required for growth, maintenance and repair. If you compress one of the hoses, such as by placing a brick on it, the normal flow of water is blocked, or at least reduced, thereby causing increased pressure in the hose and decreased water to the lawn. The heavier the brick, the greater the block, and the less water delivered to the lawn. Similarly, the more compression placed on a tissue, the less blood delivered to a muscle, which means cells in that region are deprived of essential oxygen and nutrients and will not function properly. The compressive techniques used in deep tissue massage serve as a temporary block to blood supply but have the overall effect of increasing blood flow to tissues.

Imagine stepping on a brick with your full body weight to block the flow of water in a hose. With the flow fully blocked, pressure builds up in the hose, as described. Imagine what will happen when you remove your foot from the brick *and* remove the brick from the hose. Fluid under higher-than-normal pressure suddenly surges through the hose. It is possible that this is what happens when we compress muscles during deep tissue massage. Have you noticed during massage that compressed areas quickly flush pink or red upon release of compression? When we compress tissue using our forearms, fists, elbows or a massage tool, we temporarily impede blood flow. When the compressive force is released, there is a sudden increase in blood flow to the tissues being worked, and areas that were pale prior to compression suddenly turn pink or even red. Obviously, effleurage encourages the dispersal of blood through capillaries and is thus used immediately following the administration of each compressive technique. The gentle shearing action of effleurage is useful also because it targets tissues differently from compressive techniques, which might have been administered perpendicularly.

The effect of a repeated cycle of compression-effleurage-compression makes for a kind of pumping action that helps bring fresh blood to an area that might have been slightly ischaemic to start with. A fresh supply of blood is essential for the growth, maintenance and repair of tissues.

From a practical point of view, one of the dramatic effects of compression is to reduce pain in clients with muscle tension. For example, tension commonly develops in muscles of the shoulders, neck and back when people sit in the same position for many hours at a time, and this tension is one of the main reasons people seek treatment from a massage therapist. Such muscular pain might be derived in whole or in part from a reduced blood supply to muscles when muscles are forced to maintain shortened or lengthened positions in order to support a static posture.

The kinds of compressive techniques described in this book also affect the nerve sensors within the skin and muscle, usually resulting in a palpable decrease in tension in muscles. They can thus be used to treat increases in overall tension in a muscle (such as a cramp) or to treat trigger spots—localized areas of increased tension that appear in known locations on the body, and which are palpable. Trigger spots feel tender when pressed. They often refer pain to other areas of the same muscle or to different muscles. Pain and tension in trigger spots usually dissipate to some extent with sustained compression. Look for more information on trigger spots and how to use compression to treat them in the section Establishing Your Intention on page 17 in chapter 2.

Effects of Stretch

The passive stretching described in this book helps to lengthen tissues. It might also help realign collagen fibers and untether areas of restricted fascia and muscle. Fibrosis is the formation of connective tissue in areas where it does not normally occur. Following injury, the body lays down collagen, and in some cases this reduces muscle function by sticking fibers together. By helping to realign collagen and reduce fibrosis, the stretching techniques described can be helpful in facilitating proper muscle function as part of the rehabilitative process following injury. (As with Swedish massage, none of the techniques described in this book would be used to treat an acute injury or in the postacute stage following injury.)

Deep tissue stretching techniques might also help increase joint range when range was restricted because of soft tissues. For example, if a wrist is immobilized following fracture, the flexor and extensor muscles of the wrist might shorten, along with the associated fascia of these muscles. The consequence could be a reduction in the client's ability to use his or her wrist properly, as well as his or her fingers and elbow (also affected by the flexor and extensor muscles of the forearm). Deep tissue stretching could help increase wrist, elbow and finger flexibility.

The effects of improving joint range can be profound for the client. Increasing dorsiflexion at the ankle in a client with tight plantar flexors, for example, could make a difference in whether he can walk on that foot or not. Stretching the adductors of the glenohumeral joint could help a client abduct her shoulder, thus enabling her to reach up to brush her hair when previously unable to do so. Plantar flexors commonly shorten following immobilization of the ankle (e.g., following ankle sprain or with damage to the Achilles tendon). Adductors of the glenohumeral joint shorten following immobilization of the arm caused by fracture of the humerus or forearm, or following surgery to the breast, and sometimes even in clients who simply adopt closed or protective kyphotic postures (common in the elderly). These are just some of the examples of joint immobilization that can result in tightening of soft tissues and for which deep tissue stretching techniques are useful. I'm sure you can think of many others that may affect the knee, neck and hip.

Finally, it is difficult to separate the physical effects of compression from the effects of stretch when they are combined in a deep tissue massage routine. Psychologically, deep tissue massage is calming and induces a state of deep relaxation that facilitates an overall improvement in feelings of well-being. Powerfully sedative, deep tissue massage often has a soporific effect that benefits the client.

CLIENT TALK

A client who was undergoing a long series of dental treatments came to me requesting massage to help calm him down prior to each dental session. Wracked with anxiety and apprehension, the client reported being unable to sleep the day before his dental appointment and had tried general massage, which he found was becoming less and less effective. Focusing mostly on his neck and upper back, I provided deep tissue massage the afternoon prior to his dental treatment. The client reported an induced deep relaxation that helped him get a better night's sleep.

Benefits of Deep Tissue Massage

Many claims are made regarding the physical benefits of massage, including that massage dilates superficial blood vessels, increases the rate of blood and lymph flow, reduces muscle spasm and muscle soreness and accelerates physical repair. We can explain the theoretical processes behind these kinds of physiological benefits, but it is generally acknowledged that there is a lack of sufficient scientific evidence to endorse all these claims. Lack of clear massage protocols and varying methodologies are just some of the difficulties inherent to carrying out research on this form of therapy. One of the challenges to the scientific study of massage (including deep tissue massage) is the wide variety of applications that massage may take. Effleurage and petrissage are the massage strokes commonly used in research on the subject, but the protocols for their use are rarely stipulated. However, one sympathizes with those to whom the research task falls. As anyone who has ever tried to write out a simple recipe for a friend will tell you, even a minor change in quantities, qualities or procedures can produce dramatically different results. Do you whisk the milk and then add the flour? Or add the flour and then whisk? Does it matter if you whisk while adding the flour at the same time? For how long do you whisk—a few minutes or until the flour is dispersed? What if the flour is not dispersed after a few minutes—have you added too much flour or whisked too little? It is hardly surprising that research findings for massage interventions vary. After all, with deep tissue massage, how deep is *deep*? (For further discussion, see Establishing Your Intention on p. 17 in chapter 2.)

Nevertheless, we are gradually piecing together a clearer understanding of the physiological effects of massage. Research has tended to focus on physiological parameters, perhaps because you don't have to be Einstein to know that unless you are in the hands (quite literally) of a complete sadist, receiving massage is supposed to feel good and is thus likely to increase your sense of well-being. In a world bent on evidence-based practice, it is reasonable to expect the quest for quantitative data on the use of massage in all of its forms to continue. Currently, a large body of evidence—including the beliefs and experiences of therapists who provide deep tissue massage and the clients who receive it—supports some of the claimed benefits of deep tissue massage.

Listed here are some of the benefits of deep tissue massage observed by therapists who use the technique. Also listed are benefits for therapists considering using the techniques described in this book.

Benefits for the Client

- Temporary compression of tissues might facilitate an increase in blood flow to areas that were previously ischaemic.
- Deep tissue massage is useful for improving joint range of movement, especially when stretching techniques are employed.
- Deep tissue massage helps with the treatment of trigger points.
- The stillness of the compressive techniques might facilitate acclimatization, which is useful at the start of treatment.
- Deep tissue massage might increase blood flow to an area before treatment.
- Deep tissue massage decreases tone in muscles.
- Deep tissue massage stretches muscle and fascia.
- Techniques such as stripping (p. 48) might be helpful for improving muscle function, especially when previously damaged muscle fibers have been adversely adhered with collagen.

- Deep tissue massage can assist in the treatment of cramping.
- Deep tissue massage helps address issues of muscle imbalance by helping to lengthen targeted muscles.
- Deep tissue massage is a pleasurable sensation for clients who like deep pressure.
- Some of the stretching techniques are particularly useful for clients who like to be actively engaged in their treatment (such as many athletes).

Benefits for the Therapist

- Deep tissue massage provides the therapist with an additional treatment tool; being qualified to offer deep tissue massage in addition to Swedish or holistic massage might increase a therapist's client base.
- Deep tissue massage might be a less strenuous way to apply massage because deep tissue massage relies more on body weight and leverage than on movement or strength.
- Being able to apply (all) compressive and (some) stretching techniques through clothing or a towel means the therapist can treat some clients unable to receive oil massage.
- The therapist can treat clients in offices, through clothing, perhaps incorporating and adapting some of the techniques into a chair massage routine.
- Focusing on areas of tension and avoiding bony structures helps develop palpatory skills.
- Using forearms, fists and elbows means the therapist is less likely to suffer overuse injuries of the fingers, thumb and wrist joints.
- Deep tissue massage is safer for therapists who are hypermobile in their upper limb joints.

Where and When Should Deep Tissue Massage Be Done?

Because deep tissue massage usually involves oil, it is typically performed in a private environment such as a clinic, spa, gymnasium or a client's home. Applying this kind of massage requires focus and concentration, so the therapist must feel comfortable in the massage setting. Clients should have enough time and opportunity to become fully relaxed during the procedure. Also, massage might induce a state of deep relaxation, so there should be time and space for the client to adjust following treatment. Some therapists suggest that, following a treatment, deep tissue massage clients avoid driving, operating machinery or engaging in tasks that require considerable coordination. Thus, although the dry techniques of compression can certainly be incorporated into a seated chair routine and used to treat clients at their place of work, this kind of massage is not appropriate in all workplaces. When techniques *are* incorporated into chair massage, the massage routine tends to be of much shorter duration than a Swedish massage, and the therapist does not try to induce deep relaxation. Many therapists who provide chair massage complete their treatments with a few minutes of upbeat tapotement to stimulate the client before he or she returns to work. If this is the case, using deep tissue techniques in a chair routine is fine.

As mentioned earlier in the chapter, deep tissue techniques are often used by sports massage therapists. When used by sports masseurs, the techniques are likely reserved for addressing concerns such as a reduction in joint mobility following an injury or as part of a maintenance massage between events. The techniques are unlikely to be used before an athletic activity because the stretching of muscles has been shown to reduce muscle power. After an athletic event, general massage rather than deep tissue is used because the therapist wants to assess if any trauma to tissues has occurred during the event. An exception might be when deep tissue techniques are used to treat cramping.

Closing Remarks

Now that you have an understanding of what deep tissue massage involves, its effects and benefits and where and when it may be used, you are ready to get started with using the techniques. In the next chapter you will find many useful ways to use your body weight and equipment effectively. You will also find safety guidelines to help ensure that you work with this powerful form of massage properly.

Quick Questions

1. What two main techniques for delivering deep tissue massage will you learn in this book?
2. In what five ways can you increase the sensation of pressure for a client wanting deep tissue massage?
3. Are sports massage and deep tissue massage the same thing? How do they differ?
4. Which benefits listed under Benefits for the Client and Benefits for the Therapist are most applicable to you and the clients you treat?
5. What are three conditions that make some deep tissue massage techniques suitable for a work-based chair massage routine (even though deep tissue can be sedative)?

Preparing for Deep Tissue Massage

This chapter begins with many questions. We start by asking, 'What kind of massage therapist are you?' We acknowledge the many different approaches to deep tissue massage and raise questions concerning the no-pain-no-gain approach. In this chapter you will also identify your treatment goals (for example, do you want to alleviate cramp, facilitate deep relaxation or perhaps simply practice forearm effleurage?), determine your most favourable treatment outcomes and establish the intention with which you wish to work (such as 'confidently', 'conscientiously' or 'effectively'). You will also receive advice on how to use your body and equipment safely and effectively. A section on safety guidelines provides information on important anatomical structures you need to avoid with deep tissue massage as well as safe ways to apply the techniques of compression and stretching to avoid hurting your clients. At the end of the chapter we cover frequently asked questions, address possible concerns and offer troubleshooting tips.

What Type of Massage Therapist Are You?

If you are a newly qualified massage therapist you might have realized already that learning about deep tissue massage is a useful next step in your training. If you are a therapist trained in sports massage, you might already be using some of the techniques described here and might be curious to know if there are any extra tips and tricks you could use to further enhance your massage technique. You might be reading this book with an interest in how massage and soft tissue interventions can help improve treatment outcomes for patients with musculoskeletal problems. Or perhaps you are a sports therapist with an interest in using compression and stretching techniques to facilitate rehabilitation following injury. Whatever your background and training, you can use the skills described in this chapter to help you develop your own style of treatment.

As you will discover in chapter 3 (on compressive techniques) and chapter 4 (on stretching techniques), the elements that make up deep tissue massage are simple and may be modified or combined in many ways. Like cooking, where three chefs start with the same ingredients and use them to create three different dishes, therapists using deep tissue techniques create massage treatments using combinations of skills. It is thus useful to acknowledge that different therapists have different approaches to how deep tissue massage should be used and how best to prepare for it. A common belief among some therapists is that deep tissue massage should be painful. This issue tends to divide practitioners of deep tissue massage, so let's start with it.

Some massage therapists strongly believe in a no-pain-no-gain approach to massage. This is a particularly strong view among some sports masseurs. They believe that to be effective, deep tissue massage must be painful—that it is *inherently* painful. Their argument is based on personal experience, having observed clients report improvements in the days following sometimes excruciatingly painful work to problem areas such as the iliotibial band and calf muscles. Consequently, there are now some clients who also believe deep tissue massage must be painful to be effective.

Fortunately for those of us wishing to avoid giving or receiving pain, the idea that deep tissue massage must be painful is something of a myth. As I hope you will discover from practicing the techniques in this book, there are many ways to work deeply into tissues, and there are other treatments (myofascial release, acupuncture, etc.) of treating excessively tight tissues that in some cases might be more appropriate for a client than deep tissue massage. Most therapists are altruistic in nature, with a desire to do good for their clients. Even those therapists with a brusque approach are unlikely to remain working if they do not meet the expectations of their clients at least in part. Nevertheless, dispelling the no-pain-no-gain myth is important for those of us working in the massage profession because to buy into it has three hugely negative consequences for us all.

First, believing that deep tissue massage must be painful puts off the many thousands of massage therapists who are interested in learning this form of massage but do not want to hurt their clients. These therapists might otherwise employ deep tissue massage safely and effectively without causing pain. They would have developed a useful skill with which to help treat a wider variety of clients with a wider variety of conditions. Second, the myth puts off many clients who like the idea of receiving a deeper, more firm massage but who have heard how painful it can be. Third, the myth confuses some clients who think that *all* therapists who incorporate deep tissue techniques are going to inflict pain. Perhaps these clients have received a massage treatment in the past that was painful and are reluctant to go for massage again, even with a different therapist, despite having a condition that might be usefully treated with massage.

CLIENT TALK

While teaching a sports massage course, I noticed that one of the students had severe bruising on her lateral thigh. When questioned by another student, she explained that she was a keen runner and regularly received massage to her iliotibial band, which was excruciatingly painful but which she 'knew' worked. Though somewhat weary, the runner seemed resigned to the idea that to stay in training she had to undergo massage severe enough to cause bruising. This led to a debate in class and, interestingly, although many of the students abhorred the idea, some agreed that bruising was a natural consequence of deep tissue massage and felt that if they weren't bruised their treatment was less likely to be effective.

A premise of this book is that deep tissue massage should *never* be painful, and there are good reasons to uphold this approach. If you are uncertain whether deep tissue massage should or should not be painful, ask yourself these three questions:

1. **Is it ethical?** If a treatment happens to be painful, that's one thing, but to deliberately set out to inflict pain, believing pain to be necessary—this is quite something else. Governing bodies the world over require therapists to work within a code of conduct and a code of ethics. What do your codes say about inflicting pain? Perhaps this issue is not mentioned in your codes. Should it be mentioned? Remember that we are not talking here about the kind of pain that occurs when you are first learning to massage and perhaps press a little too deeply (and quickly ease up); nor are we referring to the kind of 'grateful pain' inherent to the treatment of trigger spots. The kind of pain that some therapists believe is necessary to achieve their treatment outcomes is often prolonged and results from sharp, fast movements or the use of excessively deep pressure in which they try to mechanically force structures to lengthen. This kind of pain causes clients to wince, grit their teeth or hold their breath. It often results in bruising.

2. **Is it legal?** All massage requires consent from the client. However, pain is highly subjective, and it seems risky to agree to apply or to receive a treatment that might be painful when degrees of pain are difficult to quantify. Experienced therapists might argue that they know their clients and know how much pain they can take and how much pain is usually needed to be effective. But could there be legal implications if there is a misunderstanding between the therapist and the client (even when a consent form has been signed)?

3. **Do painful treatments really work better than techniques applied without pain?** Physiologically, pain results in the body being flooded with endorphins and an increase in muscle tension all over the body (albeit, this is temporary). Surely, increases in muscle tension are counterproductive to what we are usually trying to achieve in massage, namely relaxation and a *reduction* of tension in the muscles.

Finally, if you still firmly believe that for a treatment to be effective for some clients and to some parts of the body it must be painful, ask yourself these additional questions:

- Are you *certain* that you cannot achieve the same result without causing pain? Could it be that there are some deep tissue techniques you have not yet discovered that might enable you to achieve the same treatment outcome, or a better treatment outcome, without causing pain?

- Is there an alternative form of treatment for which you could refer your client that would have the same (or better) treatment outcome?

Establishing Your Intention

Part of the preparatory process described in this chapter involves your feeling comfortable with the idea of deep tissue massage, and with making decisions about why you want to use this form of massage and with which clients it might work well. Prior to massage it is also a good idea to identify your treatment goals and ideal treatment outcomes and to establish your intention.

Identifying Your Treatment Goals

Once you are confident with the application of deep tissue massage, you might ask yourself, 'Why do I want to use deep tissue massage for this particular client?' Your answer might be . . .

- to alleviate cramp,
- to facilitate the treatment of trigger spots,
- to improve range in a joint,
- to facilitate deep relaxation,
- to address tension in a particular muscle group,
- to overcome musculoskeletal imbalance or
- to improve posture.

These are all ways that deep tissue massage can be used to treat a specific problem. It might also be the case that you simply want to incorporate deep tissue massage into your regular massage routine for clients who like the sensation of deep pressure. When you have a specific treatment outcome in mind (e.g., an increase in the range of a joint), it is still useful to allow yourself the flexibility to respond intuitively to areas of tension you might discover during the treatment.

When using deep tissue techniques for the first time, it is helpful to practice on family and friends or colleagues. If you have this opportunity, you might want to set specific treatment goals for yourself based on how the techniques are applied.

Here are some examples of useful goals when practicing:

- To master the use of forearms on the back of the legs and thighs so that I feel confident in using this technique with my clients in prone. (For these techniques, see p. 136, Using Your Forearm on the Calf; p. 140, Using Your Forearm to Apply Soft Tissue Release; and p. 142, Using Your Forearms on Hamstrings.)
- To see if using the techniques described for tight adductors of the shoulder makes a difference to a friend's stiff shoulder. (For these techniques, see p. 152, Applying Pressure to Latissimus Dorsi; p. 153, Treating the Posterior Shoulder; p. 162, Finding the Teres Muscles; p. 163, Working the Posterior Shoulder; and p. 164, Tractioning the Glenohumeral Joint.)
- To see what happens when I provide a regular full-body Swedish massage but with my treatment couch set 2 inches (5 cm) lower than usual.
- To practice all the techniques in the side-lying position (see pp. 178-182).

Although these goals are only loosely stated and not as rigid as SMART goals (that is, goals formulated in terms of being specific, measurable, achievable, reasonable and timely), they are nevertheless useful and will enable you to reflect on your use of deep tissue massage.

Identifying Your Ideal Treatment Outcomes

What is your ideal treatment outcome? If, for example, you are using deep tissue massage to treat cramping, your obvious ideal outcome is to effectively alleviate this condition. If your goal is to facilitate deep relaxation, your ideal outcome might be for your client to report that she feels more relaxed following a deep tissue treatment than she did following a regular Swedish massage treatment.

Establishing Your Intention

Along with identifying an ideal treatment outcome, you should also establish your intentions for a treatment. Doing so helps make treatments most effective. For example, do you intend to massage in a calm yet confident manner? Is your intention to soothe and relax? Do you wish to convey an expression of care and empathy? You need not discuss your intention with your client. You are not trying to transmit your intention. Clients will respond to your intentions even when the intentions are unspoken, but your intention should be clear in *your* mind.

CLIENT TALK

When working as a corporate massage therapist, I had a regular client who was 6 feet, 3 inches (1.9 m) tall and quite muscular who liked to receive deep tissue massage once a week. One day I was exceptionally tired and wondering how I was going to perform an effective treatment for this man, who was my last client of the day. My intention was to provide the same quality of massage with half the effort I usually used. As I lowered the treatment couch I remember thinking that I had to *sink into* the muscles, which was not difficult as I leaned onto the client with my forearms. At the end of the session the client said it was the best massage he had received from me in two years. I learned a lot about the value of intention from that session.

Selecting Emotional States

Here are some terms from which to select an emotional state prior to beginning a massage treatment:

Calm	Conscientious	Grounded
Caring	Creative	Optimistic
Compassionate	Effective	Positive
Confident	Energized	Sensitive

So far we have considered how you might prepare your mind prior to massage by determining treatment goals, ideal outcomes, and your intention for the treatment. Now let's consider how best to use your body and equipment.

Using Your Body

Assuming you are in good health and feel rested and energized, there is little you need do differently to prepare yourself to apply deep tissue massage. However, you will be using your body in a way different from when you apply Swedish massage techniques, so you might find it useful to read through these guidelines relating to the use of forearms, fists and elbows.

Forearms

Using your forearms to massage means you need to get closer to your client, and it is tempting to flex at the waist to do this. You will be working with your treatment couch set at a fairly low height because this facilitates leverage. Prolonged unsupported flexion of the trunk strains the ligaments of the back, results in pain and could lead to problems later. Instead, when using your forearms, ensure you are either in a good, wide stance or that you are supporting yourself by resting your other arm on the treatment couch (or on the forearm you are using to massage). An alternative is to sit on the treatment couch, as in the example shown on page 97 under Using Your Forearm on Trapezius (With Arm Abducted). The disadvantage of sitting in this way is that you need to twist slightly at the waist to apply the stroke, and some therapists find this position uncomfortable.

Something else to consider when using your forearms is that pressure will be more concentrated to the glenohumeral joint of your own shoulder. When working statically, such as when applying compression (see, for example, p. 118, Using Your Forearm on Gluteals), this is not normally a problem. Problems occur when you start to apply forearm effleurage from a static position and do not move along the treatment couch. With the application of lighter massage this is fine, but with deeper pressure you start to both compress and move your own joint, grinding it as you pivot from the shoulder. The simple solution is to try to always move alongside the treatment couch as you effleurage, sustaining pressure through your glenohumeral joint yet minimizing its movement.

Fists

To make a fist we must flex the metacarpophalangeal joints that form the knuckles (where the hand meets the fingers) and the interphalangeal joints of the fingers (figure 2.1). When using your fists to apply strokes in deep tissue massage it is best to avoid applying pressure while these joints are unsupported. This prevents directing pressure through the joint in such a way that compromises its stability. Pressure is best directed through the bones of a joint when those bones are end to end, rather than angled with respect to each other. But to work with the bones of the hands and fingers end to end means you have your fingers straight, in the extended position, not in the shape of a fist. The most preferable way to use your fists safely is *either* to keep your fingers fairly loose, cup your hands together (e.g., the therapist's right fist on p. 112 under Fisting the Medial Calf) and press through the relatively flat surface provided by your meta-carpals, *or* you can form a tight fist and press through your proximal interphalangeal

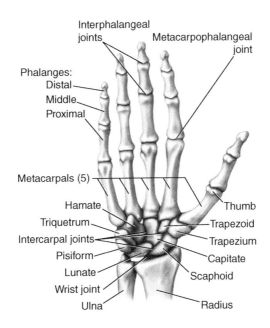

Figure 2.1 Bones and joints of the right hand, palmar view.

Reprinted from T. Behnke, 2005, *Kinetic anatomy*, 2nd ed. (Champaign, IL: Human Kinetics), 77.

joints, which should be firmly supported and unmovable in this position (e.g., p. 122, Fisting Hamstrings).

As with other joints, it is safer to keep your wrist joint in a neutral position when using fisting to apply deep tissue massage strokes. One reason therapists suffer overuse injuries is that they frequently apply constant pressure through an extended wrist joint. Wrist extension is, after all, inherent to the stroke of effleurage. Radial and ulnar deviations also occur in our wrists as we massage. Therapists risk injury to this joint when using repetitive rotary-type movements with pressure, such as when using fists to knuckle the upper trapezius. With light massage, overuse injuries of the wrist are not likely to be a problem, but as the pressure and frequency of your treatment increases you risk sustaining pain. You might also develop laxity in this joint if it is not protected.

Elbow

As when using your forearms, when using elbows it is necessary to lean onto the client, so you again need to guard your own posture to prevent injury to your back. In addition, remember that the ulnar nerve runs close to the surface of your elbow. If you experience pain, numbness or tingling in your arm when using your elbow, you might be compressing the ulnar nerve. You should stop using the technique or apply pressure with a different part of your elbow.

Tips for Using Your Body Safely

■ **Don't strain.** If after practicing you are still finding a technique difficult to apply and are unable to modify it in a way that makes it more comfortable for you, stop using that technique. Although subsequent chapters contain many tips and tricks to help you grasp the intricacies of this type of massage, we have avoided being too prescriptive in terms of exact handholds and stances. For example, you don't *have* to use your elbows for compression; you don't *have* to employ dry stretching. Like a chef using whichever ingredients he or she chooses to use, you should create the dish *you* want in developing a treatment that is unique to you. Deep tissue massage should be enjoyable for the client and should also be enjoyable for you to administer.

■ **Don't hold your breath.** When first learning deep tissue massage, therapists sometimes unconsciously hold their breath while applying compressive techniques. This might occur because (being naturally cautious and sensitive to the client) the therapist is anxious about pressing too deeply. Holding your breath increases the tone in your own muscles, and this sensation is transmitted to the client. Try to relax and make a conscious effort to breathe normally while applying deep tissue techniques.

■ **Use leverage.** When possible, make sure you are working with the best possible mechanical advantage. Sometimes lowering the treatment couch slightly, working closer to the client, or slightly adjusting the angle with which you direct your pressure can make for a significantly different effect.

■ **Listen to your body.** When you engage in a new sport or strenuous physical activity for the first time you often experience all sorts of muscular aches and pains, commonly known as delayed onset muscle soreness (DOMS). You might discover that DOMS also occurs when you are first learning to use deep tissue massage. This does not necessarily mean you are using the techniques incorrectly. But if you continue to feel muscle or joint pain, either stop using a particular technique or apply the technique differently.

Choosing Where to Use Forearms, Elbows, Fists and Squeezing

Your forearms help you provide compression or compression plus stretch to a broad area of muscle and tissue. They are thus relatively safe to use to help you apply deep tissue massage to most parts of the body. They don't work well when used on the chest (because of the bony clavicle), are not appropriate for use on the face and should be used with caution on the neck, where even broad pressure could be injurious to some structures. The forearms are seldom used without oil as part of dry stretching because this is uncomfortable to receive.

Your fists can be used simply to compress tissue but are more popularly used with oil to compress plus stretch an area. The pressure delivered with fisting is more specific than when a forearm is used but less targeted than an elbow, so the technique works well when treating the large muscles of the lower limb (such as the hamstrings, quadriceps and calf) and, with less pressure, can be safely used on the muscles of the upper limb, such as the biceps, triceps, and wrist flexors and extensors, as well as on the hands and feet. Fisting is particularly helpful for treating the iliotibial band on the lateral thigh, where the therapist can often reinforce the point of contact with the client's body by fixing his or her own elbow to their own waist (see p. 116, Fisting the ITB). Fisting is commonly used by some therapists in a knuckling type stroke to treat the upper trapezius and lateral neck muscles with the client supine. Because the pressure used here is relatively light, this technique is generally safe for the client.

Your elbows are useful when you need to compress tissues statically. Elbows are commonly used with oil to provide compression plus stretch in what is sometimes called stripping. They are seldom used without oil as part of dry stretching because this is painful to receive. The elbow works well for the treatment of small, defined areas and for this reason can be used almost anywhere on the body where you can get leverage and stabilize your point of contact, such as when the elbow is applied to the calf (see p. 137, Using Your Elbow on the Calf). Static pressure has been found useful in treating trigger spots, and use of the elbows to apply pressure to these spots is a good alternative to using fingers and thumbs. There are certain anatomical points on the body to which firm direct pressure (by any means) should be avoided. For more information, see pages 24-27. If pressure elicits pain, numbness or tingling in the lower limbs when you apply dry stretching to the piriformis muscle (p. 66), stop because this indicates you are compressing the sciatic nerve. Always avoid the no-pain-no-gain approach.

Squeezing can be used statically as a form of compression. When squeezing is used to pull muscles away from the bone (as in the example on p. 51 for the calf squeeze or quad squeeze), oil helps glide the palms over the skin. Without oil, the technique tends to be uncomfortable. Squeezing works best on muscles that can be gripped, or on the hands and feet, but it cannot really be used on flatter muscles, such as the tibialis anterior. It can be used on the forearms, but this requires gripping the forearm itself rather than the forearm muscles because these many strap-like muscles are wrapped in thick fascia and are difficult to separate from each other or from the bone during squeezing.

Using Your Equipment

The equipment used in deep tissue massage is much the same as for regular massage: a treatment couch, oil and towels. Other useful items are very small towels or facecloths, a bath sponge and tools, if you choose to use them.

■ **Treatment couch.** One of the first things you can do to facilitate deep tissue massage is to lower your treatment couch by 2 inches (5 cm). This gives you much better leverage to access the client's body, enabling you to use your body weight to lean onto the client rather than having to hunch your shoulders or go up on your toes to get over and onto the muscles.

■ **Oil.** Many of the compressive techniques, and some of the stretching techniques, described in this book do not require oil. When oil, wax, balm or cream is used you will find that you get a better grip on tissues when you apply less of it. Following the application of compressive techniques, it is necessary to effleurage and perhaps petrissage to soothe the area, in which case you need to reapply more oil.

- **Small towels or a facecloth.** It is useful to apply compressive techniques through a small towel or a facecloth because this gives considerably better grip to underlying tissues, especially when oil has previously been applied. A small towel or facecloth can also be folded and used to disperse pressure during compressive techniques. This is especially useful when working close to bony areas when you are first learning deep tissue massage.

- **Bath sponges.** Like towels, sponges are useful to press through and disperse the pressure of compressive techniques.

- **Tools.** Many great massage tools are available, but you do not need to buy expensive tools and can in fact improvise, using other objects. Ask two questions when selecting an object to be used as a massage tool: Can it be used safely? and Can it be used effectively? The answer to both questions needs to be '*yes*' before you select that object. See pages 28-29 for safety guidelines relating to the use of tools.

Understanding Cautions and Safety Issues

In the section Using Your Body you learned there are certain ways to safeguard your own body when using your forearms, fists, elbows and squeezing techniques. In this section we present information to help you apply deep tissue massage safely as it relates to the client. For convenience, the information has been grouped under three headings:

- Safety Guidelines: Anatomical Considerations—these alert you to parts of the body about which you should be particularly aware.

- Safety Guidelines: Methods of Application—these address issues relating to the application of compressive and stretch techniques.

- Safety Guidelines: Additional Contraindications and Cautions—these cover issues not included in other sections.

Note that the guidelines provided here should be taken into account in addition to the normal total and local contraindications for massage. If clients are contraindicated for general massage, in most cases they will be contraindicated for deep tissue massage. An exception might be when a client has a skin condition, such as psoriasis, in which case the use of oil might be inappropriate, but these clients could receive compressive massage through clothing or a towel.

Safety Guidelines: Anatomical Considerations

For certain anatomical structures deep tissue massage is either contraindicated or should be used with added caution.

HEAD AND NECK   As you know, the head, neck and facial muscles all benefit from massage. Deep tissue techniques to these parts of the body are not included in this book with the exception of some techniques that focus primarily on the posterior neck (e.g., p. 99, Applying Digital Pressure to the Neck Muscles; p. 91, Applying Digital Pressure to Cervical Muscles; p. 100, Applying Digital Pressure to the Occipital Region) or the large fleshy upper fibers of the trapezius muscle (e.g., p. 78, Using Your Forearm on Upper Trapezius; p. 94, Pulling Through Trapezius; p. 84, Fisting Trapezius; p. 85, Using a Tool on Trapezius; p. 101, Using Forearms With the Client Seated; p. 102, Using Elbows With the Client Seated). The techniques described to the posterior head and neck are relatively gentle because they involve massage using the fingertips. Even so, be aware of the spinous processes of the cervical spine and avoid harsh compression of the tissues there, which could cause bruising.

Techniques to the upper fibers of trapezius are safe for the neck because they do not compress important vascular, neural or lymphatic cervical structures. During massage to the upper fibers of trapezius and to the levator scapulae, pain and unusual sensations are sometimes referred to the face and head when trigger points are compressed. This is quite normal and subsides almost instantly but should be mentioned when treating clients unaccustomed to receiving deep tissue massage to these muscles. One reason that massage to the upper fibers of trapezius and levator scapulae in three-quarter lying (see, for example, p. 78, Using Your Forearm on Upper Trapezius; p. 79, Using Your Elbow on Levator Scapulae) is so effective is that the therapist has the advantage of leverage when working in this position. It is easy to compress tissues against the transverse processes of the vertebrae in this position, so caution is required.

Massage to the scalene muscles, plus to the sternocleidomastoid on the anterior aspect of the neck, is useful for lengthening or alleviating tension. Although you may not be using deep pressure, you are likely to be including treatment to these muscles in your general massage routine anyway and no doubt know to avoid pressure to the common carotid artery, which lies in this region. It is also wise to avoid deep pressure to the underside of the mandible, where there are many lymph nodes.

SHOULDERS   The main area of which to be aware when treating muscles of the shoulder is the axilla. Here you will find the nerves derived from the brachial plexus and many lymph nodes, none of which should be compressed. It is often useful to treat the teres major and teres minor muscles here, both originating on the lateral border of the scapulae. Although it is perfectly safe to compress these muscles (see p. 162, Finding the Teres Muscles, and p. 163, Working the Posterior Shoulder), be aware that this area is likely to be sensitive, especially if the client is not accustomed to receiving treatment to this part of the body. Be cautious when treating subscapularis in the supine position (e.g., see p. 156, Accessing the Lateral Border of the Scapula).

Sometimes clients experience anterior shoulder pain when receiving massage to the triceps in the supine position (e.g., see p. 154, Using Your Forearm on Triceps) because tissues of the anterior shoulder are compressed, or there might be bony impingement of the head of the humerus with the acromion process. The simple solution is to avoid sustained massage with the shoulder elevated in this way.

ARMS, WRISTS AND HANDS   Deep tissue massage to the upper limbs is safe providing you stop or reduce pressure if the massage elicits pain, tingling or numbness, because this indicates possible nerve compression. The techniques described in this book provide you with considerable leverage with which to compress tissues, so nerve compression is more likely than when applying lighter forms of Swedish massage. The technique described on page 154 (Using Your Forearm on Triceps) is a good example of where nerve compression might occur when deep pressure is applied. Be aware also that the ulnar nerve courses through the ulnar groove close to the surface of the body on the posterior elbow and can be compressed in this region.

You should avoid direct pressure into joints. The cubital fossa on the anterior elbow contains many lymph nodes (as well as nerves and vascular structures), and the carpal tunnel of the wrist houses the median nerve, none of which should be compressed. Glide over these areas with reduced pressure just as you would when providing Swedish massage.

Although not contraindicated, deep localized pressure to the thenar muscles of the palm or to the web of the thumb is quite painful for some clients. The techniques of fisting (see p. 159, Fisting the Palm) and squeezing (see p. 160, Squeezing the Palm) to this area should be safe to apply because they deliver strong but broadly dispersed pressure to the hands.

TRUNK   Muscles of the trunk can be effectively treated in supine, prone or three-quarter lying, but safety guidelines should be taken into account for each of these positions.

In supine, it is not necessary to apply deep pressure to the abdominal region. When treating the diaphragm (e.g., see p. 92, Applying Gentle Pressure Beneath the Ribs), keep pressure fairly light and directed to the underside of the costal arch. This avoids deep pressure to the liver, which could be damaging. Similarly, avoid deep pressure to the descending aorta, inferior and deep to the xyphoid process.

Also in supine, remember that pressure to the coracoid process on the anterior shoulder, though not dangerous, can be quite painful. Pain is more likely when applying the techniques shown on pages 88 (Applying Digital Pressure to Pectorals), 89 (Fisting Pectorals) and possibly 87 (Stretching Pectorals) if you happen to press on the bony structure.

When treating a client in prone position with techniques such as that shown on page 95 (Using Your Forearm on the Lumbar Region), deep pressure to the bony structures is painful, so avoid pressing into the spinous processes of the spine, spine of the scapula or directly onto the ribs. When using your elbow, as on page 98 (Using Your Elbow on Trapezius), make sure you are always on the fleshiest part of the muscle and using only light pressure over bony regions. Avoid deep pressure to floating ribs and to the kidneys.

Something else to bear in mind when treating clients in prone is that when you lean on them through your forearm you are compressing the thorax. You don't want to squash the breath out of your client but to depress their tissues, so simply avoid sustained compression.

When treating quadratus lumborum in the three-quarter-lying position (see p. 83, Using Your Elbow on Quadratus Lumborum), take care because this position allows greater access to this muscle, some parts of which might be sensitive to localized deep pressure. Try to stick to the muscle itself, avoiding pressure with your elbow directly on the iliac crest, where the muscle originates. Also be careful of the floating ribs and kidneys when using your forearms for more general strokes (e.g., see p. 81, Forearm Sweep).

PELVIS AND BUTTOCK   A couple of important structures need to be taken into account when treating the pelvic and gluteal areas. The first is the femoral triangle, an area on the anterior thigh containing the femoral nerve, femoral artery and vein, plus lots of lymph nodes. It's not usual to treat this area with deep tissue massage, but you should be aware of it, especially when applying techniques to the anterior thigh and adductors, such as those on p. 109 (Using Your Forearms on Adductors) and p. 126 (Using Your Forearm on the Quadriceps). It is unlikely that you will be working right up into the proximal adductors, but do be aware of the many lymph nodes in this area.

The second important structure to be aware of is the sciatic nerve, which is most likely to be unintentionally compressed when treating piriformis in prone (e.g., p. 145, Accessing Piriformis), and also possible when treating it in the side-lying position (e.g., p. 119, Using Elbows on Gluteals). If your treatment produces symptoms of pain, numbness or tingling in the buttocks or lower limbs, stop or reduce your pressure.

THIGHS, LEGS, ANKLES AND FEET   Focused treatment to the origins of the gastrocnemius muscle on the posterior condyles of the femur, and to the distal ends of the hamstring muscles on the proximal ends of the tibia and fibula, is often hugely beneficial. However, because of their close proximity to the popliteal space, you must take care that you are always on one of these muscles or its tendon and not pressing directly over the back of the knee when treating clients in prone, because there are many lymph nodes here, plus the femoral artery, vein and nerve. Massage to the very back of the knee is beneficial for soothing the muscles on the posterior aspect of the joint (popliteus and plantaris) but is always performed lightly and is thus not included in our discussion on deep tissue techniques.

Other interesting structures of which to be aware are bursae. These are found in many joints but are numerous in and around the knee, where they sometimes get inflamed because of overuse or sustained pressure. Resulting conditions are given popular names, such as housemaid's knee or clergyman's knee. It is likely you will be focusing deep tissue massage to the bellies of muscles rather than to nonmuscular structures around the knee joint and thus will not be treating the knee area in clients with bursitis.

As with other parts of the body, avoid localized deep pressure to prominent bony areas. The main ones to watch for in this area are the iliac crest (as when treating quadratus lumborum in three-quarter lying, as shown on p. 83, Using Your Elbow on Quadratus Lumborum); the greater trochanter of the femur when treating the iliotibial band (p. 129, Fisting the ITB) and tensor fascia latae (p. 120, Using Your Elbow on Tensor Fascia Latae); the epicondyles of the femur when treating the lateral thigh (p. 116, Fisting the ITB, and p. 117, Applying Soft Tissue Release to the ITB); and the malleoli of the ankle (p. 113 Using Your Elbow on the Medial Calf). Nerves and blood vessels are also located around the ankle, so although massage to the Achilles might be beneficial, very deep pressure to this region is inadvisable.

Safety Guidelines: Methods of Application

In this section we provide safety guidelines relating to the way in which a technique is applied rather than to which part of the body it is applied.

COMPRESSIVE TECHNIQUES   For some clients compressive techniques are not appropriate. More information about these clients can be found in the section Safety Guidelines: Additional Contraindications and Cautions on pages 29-30.

Forearms   Notice what happens when you clench your fist while using your forearm. You should discover that, for the client, the sensation of pressure increases. This might be a desired treatment outcome, and there might be some circumstances when you want to use this trick of increasing pressure without having to move or change the amount of weight you are using on the client. However, it is standard practice when using forearms (and elbows) to get into the habit of working with a loose wrist and unclenched fist. The rationale for this is that the tension the therapist experiences by clenching his or her fist could be unintentionally transmitted to the client, and this is quite different from the transmission of *pressure*. In this context (i.e., the clenched fist), tension is seen as undesirable—an increase in effort—not just the physical manifestation of pressure observable as an increase in the tone of the muscles of the therapist's forearm.

   You also need to be aware that compression feels different to the client when different parts of your forearm are used. The fleshy part of your forearm where the bellies of the wrist and finger flexors lie is relatively soft, whereas pressure from the ulnar border can feel quite sharp. This is important to remember when working on muscles that lie close to bone, such as tibialis anterior, or when treating muscles close to bony structures, such as the iliotibial band where it meets the lateral epicondyles of the femur (p. 115, Using Your Forearm on the ITB).

Fist   Although fisting is generally safe for most clients, you still need to avoid using it over bony areas.

Elbow   When compressed, trigger spots elicit feelings of slight discomfort that many clients describe as 'grateful pain', 'nice pain' or even as 'pleasurable'. With continued pressure these sensations usually dissipate within around 60 seconds. However, a lack of reduction in pain could indicate that you are pressing into something other than a trigger spot, and you should remove pressure from this spot. Whether you are using your elbows to treat a trigger spot or not, remember to always soothe the area afterwards with effleurage and petrissage.

   The undulating surface of muscles makes it difficult to fix them with a static pressure when using your elbow with oil, especially when stripping a muscle. Prevent yourself from slipping by using your other hand for support.

SQUEEZING TECHNIQUES   Few risks are associated with squeezing muscles. Note, however, that squeezing can feel incredibly deep to receive, even when it feels effort-less to apply, so always get feedback from your clients. Also, squeezing can pull on the hairs of the skin, especially when used on hairy calves, so use plenty of oil.

MASSAGE TOOLS   Being small, tools can be used almost anywhere on the body. They are best used as a dry technique, either through clothing or a towel, because this helps secure them to the region on which you are working and minimizes the risk of slipping. Use of a massage tool enables you to provide such deep, specific pressure that you need to be certain you are pressing into muscle and not into other important structures. Anatomical points on the body to which firm direct pressure (by any means) should be avoided can be found on pages 24-27. As with the use of elbows, use tools sensitively to treat trigger spots (p. 54), always soothing the area with massage afterwards.

STRETCHING TECHNIQUES   For some clients, stretching techniques are not appropriate. For more information, see Safety Guidelines: Additional Contraindications and Cautions.

Dry Stretching   Dry stretching can be used all over the body providing you take care to avoid pressing onto sharp bony areas such as the spinous processes of the spine or the medial border of the scapula. When dry stretching piriformis as described on page 66 (which also involves compression of the area), warm the area first and avoid applying too much pressure too soon. If pressure elicits pain, numbness or tingling in the lower limbs, stop immediately because this indicates you are compressing the sciatic nerve.

Tractioning   Tractioning is a safe way to help mobilize stiff joints that are otherwise healthy. Tractioning can be used on all the joints of the limbs but should not be used where a joint has been previously dislocated or on those likely to dislocate (e.g., if a client tells you he has a joint instability).

'With Oil' Stretching   Stretching can be applied all over the body, using oil to help incorporate this technique into the massage routine. If too much oil is used, it is difficult to get a grip on the skin, and the stretch is less effective; additionally, therapists sometimes try to compress tissues to facilitate the stretch, and this can be strenuous for the therapist. If too little oil is used, the client experiences pain when you pull on the hairs of the skin.

Although this kind of stretching can be used all over the body, it can be used specifically to increase joint mobility—and if used around a joint, mobility might be increased in that joint whether that was the intention or not. Thus, this technique should not be used where a joint has been previously dislocated, where joints are likely to dislocate or around unstable joints. As with compressive techniques, avoid pressing too deeply over bony points.

You will learn in chapter 4 that in some cases it is helpful to have clients participate in a stretch (e.g., p. 117, Applying Soft Tissue Release to the ITB) by actively contracting the muscle not being stretched. Performed too many times, active contraction can fatigue the muscle. If you intend to incorporate tractioning with oil stretching, be sure to read the safety guidelines for this technique on page 64.

Safety Guidelines: Additional Contraindications and Cautions

In addition to the general contraindications for Swedish massage, there are some contraindications you need to be aware of when planning to use deep tissue techniques.

- Both compressive and stretching techniques are totally contraindicated on osteo-porotic clients and on clients who bruise easily.

- Tractioning is totally contraindicated on hypermobile clients, on unstable joints and on previously dislocated joints. There is also no benefit in attempting traction-ing on a joint that has been fused by a pathological condition (e.g., ankylosing spondylitis), on a joint fused by surgery (e.g., to stabilize it) or on false joints (e.g., knee joints).

- When treating athletes, massage and stretching can decrease muscle power so it should be used cautiously in a pre-event setting. Also, deep tissue massage should not be used to treat athletes immediately following an event because there could be trauma to tissues that might be aggravated by compression and stretching.

- Use caution when treating clients who do not have contraindications for mas-sage but whom, following treatment, report unusual feelings of dizziness or disorientation; seek medical advice if necessary.

- Because of its deeply relaxing effects on some clients, deep tissue massage is not appropriate for use in all workplaces when incorporated in a chair massage routine (e.g., when a client needs to return to driving, operating machinery or engaging in tasks that might be dangerous).

Possible Side Effects of Deep Tissue Massage

- Dizziness and disorientation
- Bruising
- Feelings in muscles similar to delayed onset muscle soreness

Commonly Asked Questions and Concerns

Following are some commonly asked questions and concerns along with answers and ideas for solutions.

I'm worried that when using my forearms, fists or elbows I will not be able to feel the client properly.

It is true that you have fewer sensory receptors in the skin of your forearms, fists and elbows compared to your hands and fingertips. However, many of the techniques described in this book rely on compression. You can sense compression without using your fingertips because you have sensory mechanoreceptors in the joints of your wrist, elbow and shoulder that transmit information to the brain concerning pressure. When you compress a tissue, what you are sensing is the resistance to that pressure, and you can do this without using your hands.

I'm using all of my force, but the client says it's still not strong enough.

Deep tissue massage is not about force but technique. Read How Do You Increase the Depth of Your Massage? in chapter 1, page 7. Other possibilities are to lower your treatment couch, make sure you have adequate leverage, choose different techniques and, in some cases, use less oil. If all else fails, refer the client to another therapist.

I'm concerned about the amount of pressure some clients demand. I can deliver this amount of pressure, but surely it's not good for them?

Document your treatment outcomes and watch for negative side effects. If the client reports feeling fine and there is no bruising, you should be okay to continue. However, remember that if you are anxious during treatment, the client will sense this.

I can never seem to get into the neck muscles properly. Is it safe to do deep tissue techniques to the neck?

Not all techniques are safe for use on the neck. Refer to the section on anatomical considerations on pages 24-27.

I'm worried I might hurt my client when using deep tissue techniques for the first time.

It is good to be cautious. Follow the guidelines for the application of these techniques in chapters 3 and 4. Practice on friends, family and colleagues before using them on clients. Incorporate the new techniques gradually into your treatment.

I'm concerned I'll cause bruising and the client will never come back.

Bruising is rare when deep tissue massage is used on healthy clients who are not contraindicated for massage. Follow the safety guidelines for applying the techniques, and always combine deep tissue techniques with lighter strokes to help disperse blood and soothe tissues.

Deep tissue techniques take longer to apply than Swedish massage. I want to use them but cannot extend the treatment time.

This simply means you cannot apply all techniques all over the body in a single treatment. Be selective. Avoid the temptation to use the techniques at the same speed as you apply Swedish massage—this can cause pain and bruising.

I have a fixed height treatment couch that cannot be lowered. Can I still use deep tissue techniques?

Solutions are to change the couch, get onto the couch or do treatments on the floor or seated. You might find that you can apply some of the techniques, but not all of them; you might even discover new ways to get better leverage.

I'm concerned that with all these extra techniques my massage treatments will feel disjointed.

When you first trained in massage you might have focused on the application of one technique, practicing to get it right. Or you might have used several techniques but focused on one part of the body, such as the back or legs. Any skill takes time to acquire, and with practice you will learn to incorporate your favourite techniques into a regular massage routine.

I'm not sure which of the techniques to use, and I wonder if clients will enjoy a deep tissue massage as much as a Swedish massage.

A simple way to alleviate your concerns is for you to receive deep tissue massage yourself, perhaps from a colleague using the techniques described in this book. Judge for yourself, first, if you can tell if the therapist is using the palms or forearms to effleurage; second, judge which parts of the body different techniques feel best on.

Top Tips for Treating Clients

- Remember that tolerance to pressure varies. Clients with tense muscles are likely to feel you are exerting more pressure on them than those with less tense muscles.

- Tone in muscles usually decreases during a treatment as the client becomes more and more relaxed. This means you are able to access tissues more deeply and with less effort as the massage progresses. This is an important point because it means that towards the end of a treatment, when the client is perhaps deeply relaxed and her muscles pliable, you can compress and stretch tissues considerably and with great ease, which means extra caution is necessary.

- With subsequent treatment sessions, clients appear to become more and more acclimatized to the sensation of deep tissue massage, perhaps as their bodies get used to this form of treatment. You might discover when treating clients for the first time it is difficult to really 'get into' their muscles, even when you have a clear intention and work slowly and cautiously. Do not despair—with time, progress will likely be made. Don't struggle to achieve too much too soon. Massage is not an exact science, and different bodies respond in their own time scales. A client who has built up shoulder and neck tension by sitting at a desk for the last 10 years is going to respond differently from a client who has built up shoulder and neck tension from playing tennis for the first time in 30 years. However, if after six treatments you feel you are not making progress, it is time to examine your technique. If you are confident you are working correctly, it is worth considering referring the client to another practitioner—unless of course he is happy with your work.

- Performed more slowly than Swedish massage, deep tissue massage takes longer to administer. Try suggesting to your clients that instead of receiving a full-body treatment, they sometimes consider receiving deep tissue massage to one part of the body, such as the lower limbs, for one or two sessions. This will allow you to work in a more concentrated manner, which is sometimes warranted for the treatment of certain conditions.

- Conversely, working in a very concentrated manner on just one part of the body using deep tissue massage can feel strange for the client if this is not integrated into an overall treatment. There will certainly be times when it is not convenient to treat the whole body, and you might need to address a particular joint or group of muscles. The downside to this is that it can focus the client's attention solely to that area of the body. This is not always advisable, especially if the client is recovering from injury.

- If you enjoy the sensation of deep pressure during massage, you understand that it is frustrating to request deep pressure and then for the therapist not to check in with you to see if the pressure is deep enough, especially when it is not. We don't want to be asking our clients every five minutes how they are and whether the pressure is okay (and with regular clients you will have developed an intuitive sense of touch, so you will know this), but when using deep tissue techniques on a client for the first time you should request really clear feedback. Rather than asking, 'How's the pressure', be more specific. Ask, 'Do you want more pressure?'

- Maintain physical contact with the client. Some techniques might require you to add a facecloth and to work through it, then to remove this and soothe the area using oil. You will be using your body differently, too, sometimes leaning on your client, sometimes maybe even sitting on or supporting yourself on the treatment couch. When first learning, it is good practice to focus on always maintaining contact with your client. You will need to keep your equipment within easy reach and find new ways to move around the couch while keeping at least one hand on the client.

- Some therapists like to incorporate breathing techniques with clients to facilitate relaxation during the massage. Although some clients do not wish to take such a participatory role in their treatment, for those that do, the method is quite simple. Ask your client to exhale as you compress or stretch the tissues. Muscle tone is reduced on exhalation and increased on inhalation. Knowing this, you can use breathing techniques to facilitate deeper access to muscles.

- Avoid overworking any one area too enthusiastically. Instead, treat, move to another area and return to reassess the tissues. Often muscles relax when other areas are being treated, and you might find they do not need further work.

- Remember you can always incorporate and combine your other massage techniques (such as jostling and shaking) to facilitate a reduction in muscle tension.

Tips for Working Safely With Deep Tissue Massage

- Always follow general guidelines for the application of massage with relation to total and local contraindications.
- Follow the additional guidelines for deep tissue massage.
- Always warm the tissue first, just as you would with Swedish massage.
- Apply pressure and strokes slowly; reduce pressure slowly.
- Stop if the client reports pain.
- Avoid any techniques that you find uncomfortable to apply.
- Avoid techniques that compromise your own posture, even if they do not immediately feel uncomfortable to apply.
- Document any unusual responses from your client following treatment, such as bruising or feeling lightheaded.
- Always get feedback, especially when using deep tissue massage on clients who have not received it before.

Closing Remarks

Although you will be learning to use the forces of compression and stretch, remember that deep tissue massage is not forceful. There is growing interest among therapists in how to treat fascia, with myofascial 'release' courses offering specialist training in this area. Myofascial release involves subtle, less invasive treatment of tissues than deep tissue massage and the focus is, of course, on the fascia surrounding muscles, not on the muscles themselves, using gentle, sustained holds, glides and shearing forces rather than compression. Although you have chosen to learn deep tissue massage techniques, you might discover that you can achieve a more profound effect, perhaps with the sensation of having worked very deeply, with the application of *less* pressure rather than more. This is most likely to occur while applying the stretching techniques described in chapter 4.

Now that you have some ideas on how to prepare yourself before delivering a deep tissue massage, you can get started on learning the main techniques of compression and stretch, fully described in the next two chapters.

Quick Questions

1. What are three questions you might ask concerning the no-pain-no-gain approach?
2. What are two possible treatment goals for the use of deep tissue massage?
3. What are three possible positive emotional states you might choose as your intention prior to massage?
4. What simple thing can you do with your treatment couch to facilitate deep tissue massage?
5. What are some possible side effects of deep tissue massage?

PART II

Deep Tissue Massage
Techniques

The two main ways to apply deep tissue massage are through compressive techniques (chapter 3) and stretching techniques (chapter 4). In each of these chapters you will find information about when such techniques might be useful. You will also find safety guidelines with useful pointers to help you protect your own posture and joints while working, plus tips on how to be sure you are working both safely and effectively with your client. Use the tables provided at the end of each section to locate the step-by-step instructions for applying each technique to different parts of the body; these instructions then appear in chapters 5, 6 and 7. Working through the quick questions at the end of the chapters will help you clarify your understanding of how compression and stretch techniques are effectively performed.

Compressive Techniques

Let's begin your exploration of deep tissue massage with a description of compressive techniques and the key holds, moves and stances you need to know to apply the techniques. In this chapter you will find examples of the techniques along with tips and tricks to help you compress tissues safely and effectively. The tables provided illustrate when each of the techniques might be usefully employed to treat different parts of the body, full details of which appear in chapters 5 (the trunk), 6 (lower limbs) and 7 (upper limbs). Also presented are safety guidelines specific to the application of each technique.

Introduction to Compressive Techniques

Each of the many different ways to compress tissues affects the body in the same way. When you lean onto a client using your forearms, fists, elbows or a massage tool, and when you grip a muscle and squeeze it, you compress the tissue, temporarily impeding blood flow to that area. As you ease up, reducing the pressure, small blood vessels are no longer compressed and fresh blood floods the area. The effect of compression is to create a kind of pumping action that brings blood to an area that might have been slightly ischaemic to start with. Areas of tension subject to this form of compressive technique quickly flush pink or red.

Perhaps by affecting the nerve sensors within the muscle fibers, compression of this kind also helps to decrease tension in muscles prior to the use of deeper techniques. Therapists and clients frequently report being able to feel muscles 'letting go' during the compression of a muscle—there is a palpable reduction in tension in the tissues.

Tissues are naturally compressed when we massage. Effleurage compresses tissues broadly and lightly, and petrissage compresses more firmly. Many of the 'holding' techniques that probably form part of your existing massage routine are localized forms of compression and may be fairly deep, especially if you are using your thumbs to apply them. In the sections that follow we are going to explore techniques that require you to use body parts that you might not have used before in massage—forearms, fists, and elbows. We will also look at the value of squeezing techniques and the use of massage tools. Each of these methods of application may be modified to allow you to apply some very deep pressure while safeguarding your hands, fingers and thumbs in the process.

Forearms

You can use your forearms to compress tissues in two simple ways. First, you can simply lean onto the client at the appropriate spot, using your forearm to apply a single, static pressure. This localizes the pressure to one area and is quite specific (but less specific than when using an elbow). An advantage of using your forearm in this way is that the technique can be easily modified to suit the needs of your clients. Pressing through a broad, flat area of your forearm will obviously deliver a broader, more diffuse region of pressure than when you lean against the client using a smaller region of your forearm. Notice too that it is not just the degree of contact you use that affects the client's experience of pressure, but the *region* of your forearm you are using. For example, the ulnar border delivers quite a sharp sensation relative to pressing through the more fleshy part of your forearm where the bellies of the wrist and finger flexors lie.

Using your forearm to apply static pressure is a useful way to apply deep tissue techniques to muscles all over the body, including the trapezius and gluteal muscles in side-lying.

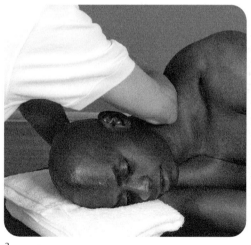
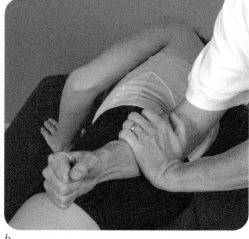

a   b

➤ See pages 78 and 118 for complete instructions on applying static pressure on *(a)* the trapezius and *(b)* the gluteal muscles.

Using Your Forearms for Static Compression

To use your forearms to apply static compression, follow these steps:

1. Identify the muscle to be compressed, focusing on the belly of the muscle. When possible, position yourself so that you can aim the force of your pressure perpendicular to the muscle belly.

2. Rest your forearm against the muscle, and slowly lean into the tissues, keeping your wrist loose and your elbow at around 90 degrees. Get feedback from your client as you do this and as you slowly increase pressure.

TIP Notice that you might need to change your stance considerably to be able to access the muscle in this way. Squatting down, or changing the direction from which you are working by just a few degrees, can make a huge difference to the amount of leverage you have.

3. Use your intuition and feedback from your client to decide when you have pressed deeply enough; remain there around 10 seconds before slowly easing up with the pressure.

4. Soothe the area either with oil or with effleurage-type strokes through clothing or a towel.

5. Repeat.

TIP Try the technique again, this time using your other forearm. It doesn't matter whether you are right- or left-handed. You will soon discover that some positions are best done always using the left or right forearm. For example, see page 109, Using Your Forearms on Adductors, and compare where your wrist falls with respect to the client's proximal inner thigh when using your left or right forearm to treat the left adductor muscles.

Another way to explore the use of this technique is to notice what happens to the sensation of pressure when you clench your fist, having already applied some pressure. Resting your left hand palm up on a table or your thigh, lean onto it using your right forearm, keeping your right wrist loose. While maintaining your pressure, clench your right fist. What happens to the sensation of pressure you feel in your left palm? For most people, the pressure increases.

Static compression using the forearm tends to be most useful when used to address localized areas of tension for which deeper techniques (using elbows and massage tools) might be too severe. Static compression is also hugely beneficial for therapists who are hypermobile in their own wrist and elbow joints and who tend to overextend these joints when applying effleurage.

The technique may be used with oil or be done dry through clothing or a towel. Not having to use oil makes this a useful technique because it means you can use it at the start of a massage treatment session, helping to facilitate muscle relaxation through the towel before you begin. This technique can also be used when treating athletes to help overcome sudden muscle spasm—because the application of localized compression reduces muscle tone in the muscle being compressed. The technique could even be incorporated into a chair massage routine for those of you providing on-site massage in offices, treating clients fully clothed.

TIP Clients with tight or bulky calf muscles often report slight discomfort when petrissage is used on this area of their bodies; they tend to be more sensitive of the contact points made by the fingers and thumbs, inherent to the application of this technique. Even when petrissage is performed smoothly and slowly, clients with tight calf muscles sometimes report sensations of pinching. For this reason, forearm massage might be preferable to petrissage for warming the calf muscle at the start of a treatment.

A further advantage of forearm compression is that it links well to another compressive technique—the use of elbows, essential for those clients who require even deeper massage.

A second way in which you can use your forearm to apply pressure is to use it with movement. One way to do this is to use your forearm to apply the effleurage stroke instead of using the palms of your hands. In response to requests for more pressure, many therapists press more firmly through their palms while effleuraging. If you have tried this, have you noticed the strain the additional pressure puts on your wrist and elbow joints? Leaning into the effleurage stroke using your forearm takes your wrist and elbow joints out of the picture and provides firm, consistent pressure, which is especially useful for covering large, bulky muscles such as the adductors, hamstrings and quadriceps, or for working into the iliotibial band on the lateral side of the thigh.

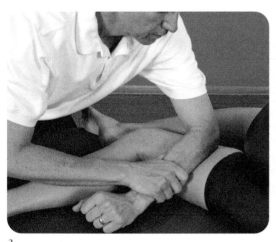   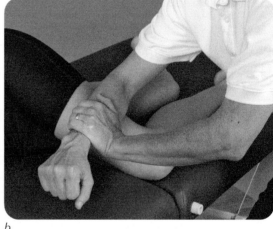

a   b

➤ See pages 109 and 115 for complete instructions on using forearm pressure with movement on the (a) adductors and (b) iliotibial band.

CLIENT TALK

I first used forearm effleurage when treating the very large and very tough hamstrings of a rugby player who wanted to feel deep pressure to his thighs during his massage treatment. Initially, no amount of deep effleurage or petrissage seemed effective, so I was forced to try something different and was relieved to discover that using my forearms to effleurage required much less effort than the techniques I had been using previously.

Using Your Forearms for Effleurage

To use your forearms to apply effleurage, follow these steps:

1. Choose a large muscle group to start, such as the adductors, hamstrings or ilio-tibial band, where you will have an opportunity to address a relatively broad surface area.

2. Starting at the distal end of the muscle, position yourself ready to lean onto the client, avoiding bony points (such as the epicondyles or the greater trochanter of the femur). This might mean taking a much wider stance than you are used to when massaging, or even leaning on the treatment couch with the other hand to support your posture.

3. Using oil, lean onto the client and *into* the tissues. Glide slowly up the muscle, from the distal to proximal ends, finishing where you feel is appropriate for your client.

TIP Fearful of causing pain, many therapists attempt forearm effleurage without actually leaning onto their clients. This makes the technique feel strenuous to apply, and of course clients do not feel they are receiving deep tissue massage. Once you are sure you are not on bony areas, intend to lean onto the client, lean onto them, and slowly perform your effleurage, supporting yourself to avoid damaging your own posture. Provided you move slowly and get feedback from the client, this is a perfectly safe technique.

4. Repeat.

As with static forearm compression, it is useful to change forearms and try the technique again, noting which forearm works best.

TIP Notice in the photos on page 40 that the therapist has chosen to reinforce his forearm using his other hand. This not only increases the pressure being used but helps stabilize the therapist's posture.

Table 3.1 shows in which chapters you can find step-by-step instructions for how to use your forearm on many different parts of the body, both statically and with effleurage.

Safety Guidelines for Using Your Forearms

As with all techniques, a couple of safety points must be taken into account. It is important that while using your forearm to effleurage you are also leaning onto the client—you are not simply using your forearm to sweep oil over the area but to apply a massage stroke designed to compress tissues. To do this requires leaning close to your client, so it is important to avoid unsupported flexion at your waist because this could strain your back. Make sure that when you apply the stroke you are either in a good, wide stance or that you are supporting yourself by resting your other arm on the treatment couch (or on the forearm you are using).

Now that you have taken your wrists and elbows out of the picture, pressure is more concentrated on the glenohumeral joint of your shoulder. Avoid grinding this joint.

Table 3.1   Situations in Which Compressive Forearm Techniques Are Useful

Chapter	POSITION		
	Three-quarter lying	**Supine**	**Prone**
5	Using Your Forearm on Upper Trapezius Using Your Forearm on Quadratus Lumborum	—	Using Your Forearm on the Lumbar Region Using Your Forearm on Trapezius
6	Using Your Forearms on Adductors Using Your Forearm on the ITB Using Your Forearm on Gluteals	Using Your Forearm on Hamstrings Using Your Forearm on the Calf Using Your Forearm on the Quadriceps Using Your Forearm on the ITB Using Your Forearm on the Adductors	Using Your Forearm on the Calf Using Your Forearm to Apply Soft Tissue Release Using Your Forearms on Hamstrings
7	Using Your Forearm on Deltoids	Using Your Forearm on Triceps	Using Your Forearm on Wrist Extensors

Grinding of the joint will occur if you remain in a static posture while performing the technique, pivoting from the shoulder. Aim to move along the treatment couch as you effleurage, moving your body in line with the stroke rather than remaining in one posture.

Advantages, Disadvantages and Uses of Forearm Compression

After practicing compressive techniques using your forearm, tick the statements with which you agree in the following three lists:

Advantages

- Easily adapted to enable the therapist to apply more or less pressure
- Easily adapted to allow the therapist to localize pressure
- Avoids strain on the therapist's wrist and elbow joints
- Is a useful alternative for warming the muscles of clients who feel petrissage to be 'pinching'
- Easily links to compressive techniques using the elbows
- Can be used with oil or as a dry technique
- Can be used through a towel or through clothing

Disadvantages

- It can take time for therapists new to forearm techniques to learn to lean onto their clients.
- Application of the technique requires the therapist to get closer to the client and requires a change in the therapist's working posture—this might take time to get used to.

When Is the Use of Forearms Indicated?

- When you want to address localized areas of tension for which the use of elbow compression or massage tools would be too severe
- When you have overused your own wrists and elbows but wish to provide massage
- When your wrists and elbows are at risk of damage through overuse or because you are hypermobile in these joints
- When you need to address cramp in a muscle
- When you wish to incorporate a compressive technique into a chair massage routine
- When you need to provide massage through clothing, such as at a sporting event

Fists

Another way to compress tissues while avoiding strain to your hands is to use your fingers cupped into a fist. This technique works well when you need to apply compression with oil to a wide strip of muscle, such as when working up the medial calf. It is a technique easily applied with deep pressure to long muscles, such as the hamstrings, or with less pressure to long muscles, such as the tibialis anterior and extensors of the wrist and fingers (see, for example, p. 146, Fisting Tibialis Anterior, and p. 165, Using Your Forearm on Wrist Extensors).

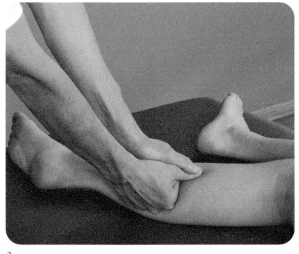
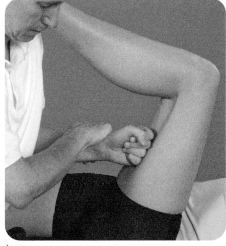

a   b

➤ See pages 112 and 122 for complete instructions on using fists to apply compression to the (a) medial calf and (b) hamstrings.

Many therapists use their fists to knuckle the trapezius muscle in a supine client, working the muscle either bilaterally or unilaterally on its upper fibers, up into the back of the neck (see p. 84, Fisting Trapezius). The disadvantage here is that it is tempting for the therapist to use a rotary-type movement at the wrist as he applies pressure. Although this feels delightful for the client, it is not particularly good for the therapist's wrist joint.

It is best to perform fisting with the arms held straight out in front of you. This means keeping your wrists in a neutral position (neither flexed nor extended) while keeping your elbows extended. This can be tricky, especially if you are hypermobile and tend to overextend your elbows when trying to keep them straight. Working through a forearm, you can easily learn to relax and lean into the tissues, whereas this technique requires effort to maintain proper alignment in your own joints, and the risk is that you transmit this sensation of effort to your client. However, the use of fists does have a place in deep tissue massage, fitting better to some parts of the body than to others. Fisting is also useful for strong therapists with large forearms, fearful of leaning too heavily onto their clients. Therapists unable to maintain strong wrist alignment can apply the technique single-handed, using their other hand to support the fist being used (as shown in the photo on page 129).

Using Your Fists to Apply Static Compression

To use your fists to apply static compression, follow these steps:

1. Identify the muscle to be treated and position yourself at its distal end.
2. Cup your fists and, avoiding pressure to bony areas, lean gently onto the client, compressing the tissues. Try to keep your elbows and wrists in a neutral position.

TIP Purists insist that this technique must be performed with the therapist maintaining wrists and elbows in a neutral position. This does indeed protect these joints from compressive forces, but in reality it is extremely difficult to maintain. As you glide over bony areas and follow the contours of your client's muscles, you will naturally need to flex both your wrists and elbows.

3. Using oil, continue to lean onto the client as you slowly glide up the muscle towards its proximal insertions, getting feedback from your client.
4. Repeat.

In an attempt to maintain wrists and elbows in a neutral position, some therapists hunch their shoulders, causing tension and pain in the upper trapezius and levator scapulae muscles. Generally, you need to set your treatment couch lower than usual to perform this compressive technique.

Table 3.2 shows in which chapters you can find step-by-step instructions for using fists on the most appropriate parts of the body.

Variations in Fisting Technique

When fisting, subtle changes in how you apply the technique can have a large impact on how it feels to receive. For example, you might choose to press through your metacarpals, keeping the proximal phalanges flat against the skin as you glide your fingers over the

Table 3.2   Situations in Which Compressive Fist Techniques Are Useful

| Chapter | POSITION | | |
	Three-quarter lying	Supine	Prone
5	—	Fisting Trapezius Fisting Pectorals	—
6	Using Your Fists on Adductors Fisting the Medial Calf Fisting the ITB	Fisting Hamstrings Fisting the ITB	Fisting the Calf Fisting Tibialis Anterior Fisting the Foot
7	—	Fisting Triceps Fisting Biceps Fist Wrist Extensors Fisting the Palm	—

muscle, as shown in the photo on page 138. Or you might decide to add some ridge-like pressures. For this second method, simply angle the position of your hand so that you are running your proximal interphalangeal joints against the muscle rather than against the flat phalangeal bones. If you keep a tight fist this technique is safe for these joints.

Safety Guidelines for Using Your Fists

In addition to following general guidelines for deep tissue massage, it is helpful when fisting to avoid pressing through the proximal interphalangeal joints while your fist is loose. Either keep your fingers fairly loose, cupping hands together as shown in the photo on page 116, or use one hand to support the wrist of the other, as shown in the photo on page 129, pressing through the relatively flat surface provided by your phalanges. Alternatively, you can form a tight fist and press through your proximal interphalangeal joints, which should be firmly supported and unmovable in this position.

Advantages, Disadvantages and Uses of Fisting

After practicing compressive techniques using your fist, tick the statements with which you agree in the following three lists:

Advantages

- Useful for applying pressure with oil to a wide strip of muscle
- An alternative technique for therapists with large forearms who are fearful of applying too much pressure to a client of disparate body size
- May be easily modified to alter the client's sensation of pressure
- Not necessary to lean close to the client to perform the technique

Disadvantages

- It can be difficult to maintain wrists and elbows in neutral alignment.
- It can be tempting to use rotary-type movements when using the wrists on the upper trapezius in supine.
- Generally, the treatment couch needs to be much lower than usual to perform this technique.
- Therapists new to the technique tend to hunch their shoulders, causing strain in the upper trapezius and levator scapulae muscles.

When Is the Use of Fists Indicated?

- When you wish to apply compressive techniques with oil to long muscles
- When you have large forearms and wish to avoid deep pressure effleurage through your palms while treating a smaller client

Elbows

Elbows are commonly used as part of a deep tissue massage routine. They can be used in two ways. First, they can provide localized static pressure to relatively small muscles that require deep pressure (such as the tensor fascia latae or levator scapulae) or to a small, specific area of a large muscle (such as the origins of the hamstrings). Second, they can apply what is sometimes called stripping—that is, the slow, continuous application of pressure with oil along a narrow band of tissue.

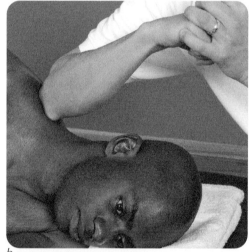
b

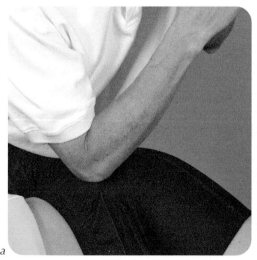
a

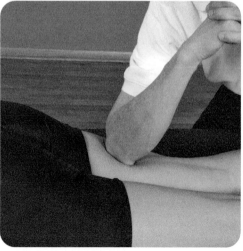
c

➤ See pages 120, 79 and 143 for complete instructions on using the elbow to apply pressure to *(a)* the tensor fascia latae, *(b)* the levator scapulae and *(c)* the hamstrings.

Covering a smaller surface area, the pressure facilitated by the use of elbows is deeper than when using forearms or fists—and might even be as deep as when using a massage tool. For this reason, it is best to use elbows for deep pressure only after tissues are thoroughly warmed. (Of course *all* deep tissue techniques have a more profound effect and are safer to apply after tissues have been warmed using regular massage techniques.)

Using Your Elbows to Apply Static Compression

Use your hand to practice this technique on yourself before trying it on a client.

1. Identify the spot you wish to treat and touch it with your elbow, keeping your elbow flexed *(a)*.

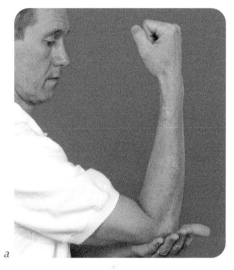

a

2. Extend your elbow slightly, while still touching the spot, *but do not add any pressure yet (b)*.
3. With your elbow on this same spot, still extended, lean onto the client *(c)*.

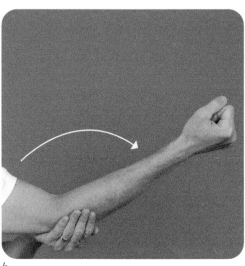

b

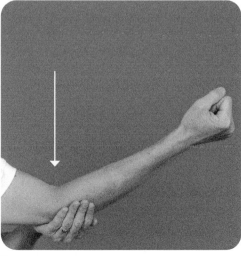

c

4. Maintaining the pressure, *slowly* flex your elbow *(d)*.

5. Ease up, reducing your pressure, and soothe the area.

6. Repeat.

TIP Notice that by changing the degree of flexion in which you hold your elbow by just a few degrees, you produce a disparate increase in the sensation of pressure reported by the client.

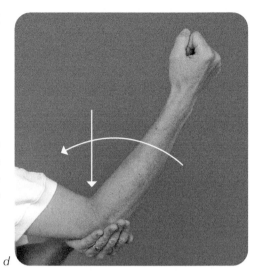

d

Using Your Elbows to Apply Stripping

To use your elbow to apply a stripping technique, follow these steps:

1. Starting at the distal end of a thoroughly warmed muscle, identify the line of tissue along which you wish to strip (e.g., the centre of the calf muscle).

2. Place your elbow at the distal end of this line, supporting your elbow with the web of your other hand.

3. Lean onto your client with your elbow and, using the guide hand, slowly move from the distal end of the muscle to the proximal end.

4. Soothe the area with strokes such as effleurage or petrissage.

5. Repeat.

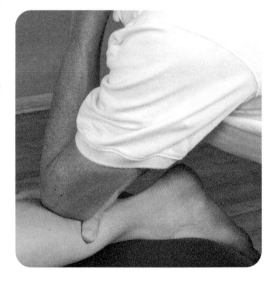

Table 3.3 shows in which chapters you can find step-by-step instructions for using your elbows on different parts of the body.

Table 3.3   Situations in Which Compressive Elbow Techniques Are Useful

	POSITIONS		
Chapter	**Three-quarter lying**	**Supine**	**Prone**
5	Using Your Elbow on Levator Scapulae Using Your Elbow on Quadratus Lumborum	—	Using Your Elbow on Trapezius
6	Using Your Elbows on Adductors Using Your Elbow on the Medial Calf Using Elbows on Gluteals Using Your Elbow on Tensor Fascia Latae	Using Your Elbow on the Quadriceps Applying Your Elbow to Tibialis Anterior	Using Your Elbow on the Calf Using Your Elbows on Hamstrings
7	Treating the Posterior Shoulder		Working the Posterior Shoulder Using Your Elbow on Infraspinatus

Safety Guidelines for the Use of Elbows

Additional safety guidelines for using the elbows relate to the fact that the pressure applied is so localized. When using the elbows, you must never compress main vascular structures, lymph nodes or nerves. You need to take extra care in controlling this technique. Be especially careful when using oil—you must guide your elbow to prevent it from slipping, keeping the elbow in the correct position on the muscle.

When using elbows to treat trigger spots, be sure to remove the pressure if the sensation of slight discomfort at the spot does not dissipate within 60 to 90 seconds. If the discomfort does not dissipate, this could indicate you are pressing into a spot other than a trigger spot.

Finally, remember that elbows should be used only after tissues have been thoroughly warmed. That said, with practice, many therapists become expert at applying just the right amount of pressure with the elbows, using this very pressure as part of the warm-up. Using elbows certainly facilitates the application of deep pressure, but such pressure doesn't *have* to be deep.

Advantages, Disadvantages and Uses of Elbows

After practicing compressive techniques using your elbows, tick the statements with which you agree in the following three lists:

Advantages

- Facilitates the application of very deep pressure
- Can be localized to a very specific spot
- Avoids strain on the therapist's wrist
- Easily links to compressive techniques using forearms
- Can be used with oil or as a dry technique
- Can be used through a towel or through clothing

Disadvantages

- Cannot be used on all muscles
- Can take time for therapists to learn to lean onto their clients when using elbows

When Is the Use of Elbows Indicated?

- When you need to apply very deep, localized pressure and do not have massage tools available and do not wish to use your fingers and thumbs
- For the treatment of trigger spots
- When your wrists and elbows are at risk of damage through overuse or if you are hypermobile in these joints
- When you wish to incorporate a compressive technique into a chair massage routine
- When you need to provide massage through clothing, such as at a sporting event

Squeezing

The simple act of squeezing tissues helps promote blood flow to the tissues in much the same way as when using forearms to apply static pressure. Compression momentarily impedes blood flow to the area, after which pressure is released and blood returns. Petrissage requires single-handed gripping and squeezing movements that can lead to overuse syndromes in the flexor and extensor muscles of the forearm, as well as overuse of the thumb. So it is useful for therapists to have an alternative to this technique. Squeezing enables you to use your shoulder adductor muscles as well as your hands to provide compression. Squeezing can be used statically but feels better to receive when combined with oil, and although it can be used on the quadriceps (p. 127, Quad Squeeze) and hands (p. 160, Squeezing the Palm), it is most commonly used on the calf.

Using Squeezing on the Calf

Squeezing may be performed with the client either prone or supine after oil has been applied to the calf.

1. Sitting close to the client with his or her knee flexed, cup your hands around the distal end of the muscle.

2. Working from the part of the muscle closest to the tibia—the deeper part of the muscle—slowly grip the tissue.

3. Maintaining your grip, allow your hands to slide off the muscle, dragging it away from the tibia.

4. Choose another, more proximal spot on the muscle, and repeat.

5. In this manner, work your way from the distal to proximal ends of the muscle. Notice how it feels to grip the main bulk of the muscle at its belly, compared with the thinner and less fleshy part near its junction with the Achilles.

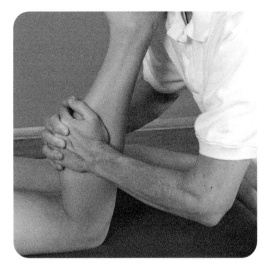

➤ See page 141 for complete instructions on using squeezing on the calf.

When treating the hands of clients, many therapists commonly use their own thumbs to apply circular pressures into the thenar and hypothenar eminences of the client's palm. Although this feels pleasurable for the client, it does not provide particularly deep pressure (because most clients do not require deep tissue massage to their hands) and is potentially damaging to the therapist's thumb. When treating clients who do require deeper massage, try compressing the fleshy thenar and hypothenar eminences in a similar manner to that described here for the calf.

Table 3.4 shows which chapters to consult for step-by-step instructions on squeezing.

Safety Guidelines for the Use of Squeezing Techniques

Squeezing is one of the safest compressive techniques, with relatively few risk factors. The main consideration is that squeezing can be deceptively deep, so be sure to get feedback from clients when first practicing this technique.

Table 3.4   Situations in Which Compressive Squeeze Techniques Are Useful

	POSITION		
Chapter	Three-quarter lying	Supine	Prone
5	—	—	—
6	—	Calf Squeeze Quad Squeeze	Calf Squeeze
7	—	Squeezing the Palm	—

Advantages, Disadvantages and Uses of Squeezing

After practicing squeezing techniques, tick the statements with which you agree in the following three lists:

Advantages

- Facilitates the application of very deep pressure (to the calf muscles, especially)
- Provides an alternative to petrissage
- Allows therapists to use their shoulder adductors in addition to wrist and finger flexors, thus reducing the likelihood of overuse syndromes
- Is easily combined with oil

Disadvantages

- Cannot be used on all muscles
- Can be difficult to use on large, hypertonic muscles, especially if the therapist has small hands

When Is the Use of Squeezing Indicated?

- When you need an alternative to petrissage for use on the calf
- When you need to apply deep pressure to clients with large, powerful hands

Tools

Now let's consider how massage tools are used to safely compress tissues. Many therapists are intrigued by the use of massage tools but often buy them and then don't know how best they should be used. Fearful of not using them correctly, they might discard the tools and revert to using fingers and thumbs instead. Using fingers and thumbs as part of a gentle Swedish massage is tolerable—and in fact essential when treating some parts of the body, such as the face—but they should *never* be used to apply deep tissue massage. Therapists who start working with clients requiring deep tissue massage sometimes fall into the habit of using their fingers and thumbs and thus suffer symptoms of overuse. Learning to use tools safely helps prevent you from sustaining overuse in your hands and allows you to apply deep tissue massage more effectively to some parts of the body. Though the tools cannot be used to treat all muscles, they are excellent for applying very deep static pressure to small, specific areas. They can be used without oil, through clothing, but work best when the area that has been treated can be soothed with strokes such as effleurage and petrissage.

Types of Massage Tools

Many types of massage tools are on the market today. You can also use some everyday items as massage tools.

1 Tennis-type balls from a pet shop
2 Index knobber
3 Child's wooden skittle from a thrift shop
4 The knobble massage tool
5 Plastic jacknobber
6 Wooden 'mouse'

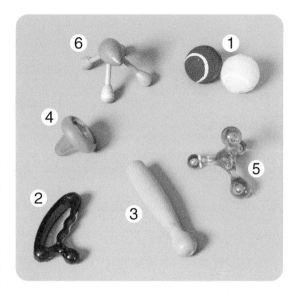

One of the most effective and least expensive tools you might use for compression is a simple tennis-type ball available from a pet shop. Designed for dogs with strong jaws, these balls are much harder than regular tennis balls; when used in treatment, they are placed beneath the client so that his or her body weight facilitates the compression. The balls work well with the client in supine position, when pressure is needed on muscles such as the upper trapezius, rhomboids or levator scapulae muscles. Although you will need to assist clients in positioning the ball against the part of their muscle that feels best, no effort is required from you to apply pressure to the area. Balls of smaller diameter can be used but tend to get lost in the padding of the treatment couch, resulting in minimal compression.

To compress tissues such as the supraspinatus muscle or the upper fibers of the trapezius with the client prone, tools such as an index knobber are useful. When using a knobber, you will probably need to sit or kneel, or to adopt a posture with a very wide stance, to get good leverage. You should keep your wrist in a fairly neutral position.

Using Tennis-Type Balls to Apply Compression

To use a tennis-type ball to apply compression, follow these steps:

1. With the client in supine position, place the ball so that it presses against that part of the muscle the client reports as feeling most beneficial. Avoid pressure to the ribs, the vertebrae and the medial border of the scapulae. Remove your hand.

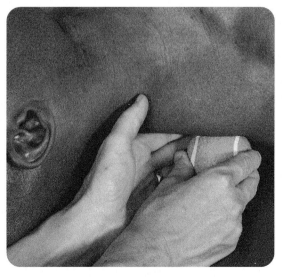

➤ See page 86 for complete instructions on using a tennis-type ball on the upper trapezius.

2. Encourage the client to relax onto the ball for no more than 60 seconds.
3. Reposition the ball to a different area and repeat.

Avoid overworking the area, using the ball to apply compression for up to a minute maximum. Ideally, it is best to soothe the area using effleurage following compression, but this means turning the client prone in this example.

TIP   Sometimes it helps if clients help position themselves over the ball, moving slightly on the treatment couch until the correct spot is reached. In this method, simply hold the ball stationary as the client gets comfortable.

Using an Index Knobber to Apply Compression

To use an index knobber to apply compression, follow these steps:

1. Locate the spot you wish to compress and place a towel or facecloth over it. Be sure you are on muscle tissue and not over bone or other vital structures such as blood vessels, lymph vessels or nerves.

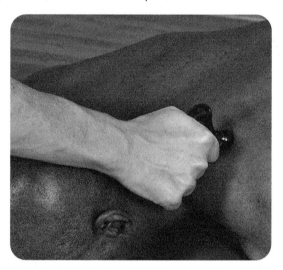

➤ See page 161 for complete instructions on using an index knobber to apply compression.

TIP   Applying oil and then placing a small towel or facecloth to the area helps ensure you will not slip while using the tool. It is tempting to apply the tool straight to the skin, but this is much harder to control.

2. Place your massage tool on the spot (*over* the towel or facecloth).
3. *Slowly* start to apply pressure, perpendicular to the muscle when possible and getting constant feedback from your client.
4. Using your intuition, and with feedback from your client, maintain deep pressure for up to 30 seconds and then *slowly* release.
5. Soothe the area using effleurage or petrissage when possible.
6. Repeat if necessary.

Table 3.5 shows in which chapters you can find step-by-step instructions for using massage tools.

Safety Guidelines for the Use of Massage Tools

Massage tools let you provide pressure as deep or deeper than when using your elbows. The area being compressed is even more specific than when using your elbows, so you need to ensure you are pressing into muscle and not into other vital structures. If you are in doubt, refer to the general safety guidelines for applying deep tissue massage, covered in chapter 1 (p. 24). As a therapist, you will be accustomed to helping clients identify 'grateful' pain, that feeling of pleasurable discomfort associated with the release of tension in very tight muscles. Of course, should your client report *pain* at any stage of the application, you should stop immediately.

Advantages, Disadvantages and Uses of Massage Tools

After practicing compressive techniques using massage tools, tick the statements with which you agree in the following three lists:

Advantages

- Facilitates the application of very deep pressure
- May localize pressure to a very specific spot on the muscle being treated
- Avoids strain on the therapist's fingers and thumbs
- Can be used with oil or as a dry technique
- Can be used through a towel or through clothing

Disadvantages

- Not suitable for all muscles (such as muscles in the face)
- Can take time to gain confidence with applying the technique
- Requires a change in working posture to gain proper leverage

Table 3.5   Situations in Which Compressive Tool Techniques Are Useful

Chapter	Three-quarter lying	Supine	Prone
		POSITION	
5	—	Using a Tool on Trapezius Using a Tennis Ball	—
6	—	Using a Tool on the Foot Treating Tensor Fascia Latae With a Tool	—
7	—	—	Accessing Supraspinatus

When Is the Use of Massage Tools Indicated?

- When you need to apply very deep, localized pressure and do not wish to use your fingers and thumbs
- For the treatment of trigger spots
- When your fingers and thumbs are at risk of damage through overuse or because you are hypermobile in these joints

Closing Remarks

In this chapter we have focused on compressive techniques, one component of deep tissue massage. In the next chapter you will find information on an equally important component of deep tissue massage: stretching.

Quick Questions

1. When using forearm techniques, what happens to the client's sensation of pressure if you clench the fist of the forearm you are using?
2. What is one of the difficulties inherent to the application of fisting techniques?
3. In addition to leaning more heavily onto the client, how can you increase pressure when using your elbow?
4. How should you prevent your elbow from slipping when using the elbow to apply a stripping technique?
5. Of all the techniques described in this chapter, which works best to apply broad, relatively diffused compression? Which works better for treating small, specific spots?

Stretching Techniques

Now that you understand how compression can be used in a deep tissue massage treatment, let's add an additional component—the stretching of tissues. In this chapter you will learn the best ways to incorporate stretching into your massage, the parts of the body to which stretching is suited and lots of tips to help you develop this skill effectively. As usual, there are also safety guidelines you need to be aware of. Tables throughout the chapter guide you to the correct chapter—chapter 5 on the trunk, chapter 6 on the lower limbs or chapter 7 on the upper limbs—to find information specific to the application of stretching to different parts of the body. Finally, you can use the quick questions at the end of the chapter to test your understanding of incorporating stretching techniques into a massage treatment.

Introduction to Stretching Techniques

Whenever you massage you stretch tissues. Unless you are using minimal pressure and large amounts of oil, even the gentlest of effleurage stretches the skin. Here we are going to look at how stretching can be incorporated into your treatment. This is not the kind of stretching you might do in the gym after a workout, or the kind of stretching you might provide for a client as a specific treatment modality (e.g., gross passive stretching or specialized forms of stretching, such as muscle energy technique or proprioceptive neuromuscular facilitation, known as MET and PNF, respectively). Nor does this stretching incorporate the kinds of active stretching you might provide for your client for use at home as part of an aftercare package. The stretching you will learn here is stretching *specific* to the application of deep tissue massage. It is frequently performed passively, by the therapist, seamlessly incorporated into the massage treatment. However, you will also learn how the client can help facilitate a stretch by contracting the muscle opposite (the antagonist) to the one you are working on, thus reducing tone in the muscle being treated (the agonist).

Stretching is inherent to almost all massage. However, the techniques used in deep tissue massage can be broadly categorized as 'without oil', or dry stretching, and 'with oil' stretching. To each of these categories we can add two elements to enhance the stretch. First, we can gently traction a limb, pulling it as we massage. Second, we can move the joint (affected by the muscles we are treating) in such a way that these muscles are stretched. Mobilizing the joint like this is performed while continuing to massage. Finally, we can add together these two elements of traction and joint mobilization, performing them at the same time, whether or not we are using oil. It is useful to note that with each subsequent additional technique—first dry stretching, and then with added traction, and then with added joint movement, and then with added traction plus joint movement—the tissues are stretched to a greater degree. Simultaneously, the client is likely to sense the depth of massage increasing. So, although performing most of these techniques without oil is possible and might benefit those clients who crave exceptionally deep tissue massage, most clients will find the techniques much less comfortable to receive than when oil is used. Some therapists might also argue that without the use of oil these techniques are also harder to 'link', making it more challenging to provide a comprehensive treatment. Here we have described the use of dry stretching techniques only where they are most useful, with the majority of add-on techniques appearing in the 'with oil' section.

Without Oil (Dry Stretching)

Most clients prefer a particular massage stroke and a particular depth of pressure and might request that you spend more time on one part of the body than another. Although we try to avoid overworking any one area, therapists instinctively gravitate to those tissues that require more focused treatment. If you have ever found yourself doing this, you might have noticed that not only does the depth of your pressure sometimes increase, but that the strokes you are using squeeze and stretch the tissues in a more concentrated way. It is to these areas of the body that dry stretching can be particularly helpful. Which areas these are depends on the needs of the client and where their fascia and muscles are most tight.

Dry techniques can be incorporated with oil at any stage of the massage treatment by simply applying the stretch through a towel or facecloth placed over the area. When used this way, dry techniques are very powerful, so caution is called for; the techniques are not appropriate for clients with fragile skin or those who dislike deep tissue treatment. Conversely, these techniques are ideal for enhancing the sensation of deep pressure and are particularly helpful when treating a muscle or area of tissue you have identified as being tight or shortened. Used in their pure, dry form, they are useful when oil might not be appropriate or might be problematic—when treating clients with psoriasis, for example. They are easy to apply, requiring little effort from the therapist, and easily modified to enhance the sensation of deep tissue massage.

In the next sections, we will look at a couple of dry stretch techniques, as well as using traction with dry stretching.

Dry Stretch

A good example of an area in which dry stretching works well is the back. The technique is easy and safe to practice in this area, and by later adding oil and applying the technique through a towel, you will quickly learn how dry stretching helps facilitate the sensation of deep tissue massage without needing to apply deep pressure.

Many therapists learn to massage the back longitudinally, sweeping their effleurage from the neck to the sacrum or from the sacrum to the neck, depending on how they have been taught to stand with relation to the treatment couch. After warming the muscles, therapists often work 'up' or 'down' the erector spinae muscles with more focused stripping-type techniques or using small circular movements. Working transversely across the back without oil stretches the skin, fascia and associated muscles away from the spine and is thus a useful addition to these techniques.

Applying Dry Stretch to Erector Spinae Muscles

Practice this technique before you have applied any oil to your client. For this technique, you always work the erector spinae muscles on the opposite side of the client to which you are standing. In other words, if you are standing to the right of the client (as in the photo), you will be working his or her left erector spinae muscles. It doesn't matter which side of the client you treat first. However, to help you grasp the technique, we start here with treatment to the client's left erector spinae muscles.

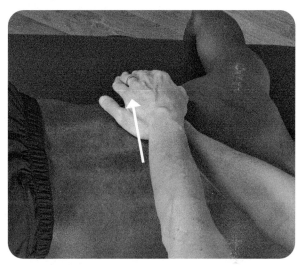

1. Stand at the right side of the treatment couch and identify the spinous processes of the client's spine. You are going to avoid pressure to these.

➤ See page 93 for complete instructions for using dry stretch on the erector spinae muscles while standing on the opposite side of the client.

2. Locate the erector spinae muscles running longitudinally down the left side of the client's back. With your hands positioned as shown, place your thenar and hypothenar eminences against the skin, over the muscles.

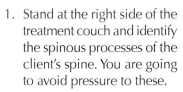 It doesn't matter whether you start close to the cervical, thoracic or lumbar spine. However, when first learning the technique, a good place to start is around the upper thoracic region; you then work towards the sacrum.

Your aim is to gently push the erector spinae muscles (and the associated tissues) away from the spine. Lock onto the tissues and gently ease them away from the spine. Keeping your elbows extended, avoid letting your hands slide across the skin. You want to stay locked to the skin and to stretch the tissue under your palms rather than gliding across it. Sometimes using a gentle rocking motion as you push the muscles away from the spine helps the client relax.

3. Work up and down the spine two or three times, *always* on the same side of the spine. It doesn't matter if you start at the top of the thoracic spine and work your way down to the sacrum, stop and return to your start position before repeating, or if you start at the thorax, work down to the sacrum and then work back up to the thorax.

TIP Notice that because of its natural lordosis and small area it is difficult to position the pads of your palms on the extensor muscles of the neck. If you want to apply the technique to this area, simply use the pads of your fingers instead of your palms. In this position (prone), it is difficult to fix these muscles in order to dry stretch them. You might find that treating them works better when you later add oil and apply this technique through a towel.

4. Once you have worked along the left erector spinae, move to the left side of the treatment couch and repeat the technique on the muscles of the client's right side.

Four Modifications to Dry Stretch the Erector Spinae Muscles

There are four ways to enhance your understanding of how dry stretching might be a useful addition to your massage skills. First, practice the technique, paying particular attention to which areas of the back seem less pliable and stretch less. Are there differences in the client's left and right sides? Is one part of the lumbar region less pliable than another? Does the technique cause the client to report sensations of 'stiffness', 'tension' or 'relief' specific to a certain area? One of the values of a dry stretching technique is that both you and your client become more aware of localized areas of tension, areas where there is *less* stretch in tissues.

A second thing you can do is notice what happens when you apply the technique through a towel, having added a small amount of oil to the client. To do this, simply effleurage the client as you might normally, with perhaps a little less oil, and then repeat the above steps through a towel. Notice that working through a towel allows you to get a better grip on the skin as the tiny fronds of the towel soak up the oil, forming a lock between the towel and the client's skin. In this manner you need apply very little pressure at all and yet are able to stretch tissues easily. Ask your client how this second method of application feels. Many clients report that it feels much more powerful, more 'deep'.

TIP If you are anxious about pressing onto the spinous processes of the spine, use one hand to locate the processes and keep that hand there as a guide; then use the other palm to stretch the tissues.

A third thing you can do is to practice the technique in different directions, all over the back, without oil on dry skin or through a towel following the application of a little oil. The step-by-step instructions on page 93 describe how to work transversely across the erector spinae muscles. However, you can work longitudinally over these muscles, or in any direction you choose. You don't have to stay on the erector spinae muscles but may choose to apply the technique to any part of the back. Use the technique on those areas that require stretching, and avoid muscles that already feel pliable or are likely to be lengthened and weak because of the posture of your client. Remember that erector spinae muscles are designed to keep us erect, and during daily activities they rarely get rest. These muscles are naturally strong in healthy individuals, which does not mean they require stretching. The middle fibers of the trapezius and the rhomboid muscles are also often long and weak, especially in clients with kyphotic postures. Stretching these muscles (using *any* stretching technique) is not necessarily helpful. Use of dry stretching to the erector spinae muscles has been described here simply because it is an easy way to learn the technique, and for the treatment of some clients it will certainly be valuable. After learning the technique, modify it to suit your needs.

Finally, notice what happens when the client receives the technique with arms in varying positions. If you apply the technique with the client prone, with arms at the sides, this feels quite different (both to give and to receive) compared to what clients feel when they abduct their arms to 90 degrees, allowing their arms to hang over the treatment couch, or even when they take their arms above their heads. Changing the position of the arms changes the position of the scapulae, which in turn affects the tension in the tissues of the back. You might discover that areas that felt relatively slack are suddenly subject to more tension. For example, if you position the client prone with arms above the head, you stretch the thoracolumbar fascia slightly. Dry stretching the lumbar area in this position aids those clients whose lumbar erector spinae or quadratus lumborum muscles are tight. However, in this position, fascia of the upper trapezius is shortened, making it harder for you to access this area with the dry stretch technique. Treating clients with tight upper trapezial fibers might be more effective when their arms are at their sides. Having the option to change the position of the client's arms in this way is useful for enhancing dry stretching.

TIP   Dry stretching may be used all over the body, following the guidelines on page 93, where dry stretching to the erector spinae muscles is used as an example.

Safety Guidelines for Dry Stretching the Back

Always work away from or parallel to the spinous processes of the spine, avoiding pressure towards or directly on the processes themselves. Similarly, avoid stretches that require you to press up and onto sharp bony ridges, such as the medial border of the scapula. Remember that ribs curve outwards and what some therapists perceive to be hardened muscles or 'knots' in muscles might actually be underlying bone. Avoid all forms of dry stretching when treating clients with fragile skin.

Finally, note that dry stretching is not limited to use on the back. You can use the technique on any part of the body, remembering to avoid pressure into bony areas and focusing the stretch to those areas you have identified as feeling most tight.

Advantages, Disadvantages and Uses of Dry Stretching

After practicing dry stretching, tick those statements with which you agree in the following three lists:

Advantages

- A stretch might be localized to a particular area of tissue.
- Dry stretching can be useful when the use of oil is not appropriate or is problematic.
- It is easy to apply.
- It can be used anywhere on the body.
- It requires little effort from the therapist.
- Dry stretching is ideal for clients who require the sensation of exceptionally deep tissue massage.

Disadvantages

- Dry stretching can be difficult to link to other techniques without the use of oil.
- It might be uncomfortable for some clients to receive.
- It is not appropriate for clients with fragile skin.

Situations When Dry Stretching Is Indicated

- When treating a muscle or area of tissue you have identified as being tight or shortened (usually used when you need to stretch a localized area of tissue)
- When treating a client who requires or values the sensation of exceptionally deep tissue massage

Traction

The use of gentle traction is an invaluable component of deep tissue massage. Traction involves gently pulling on a limb, distracting a joint and thus stretching the associated tissues. Although traction can be incorporated into an oil massage, it is best performed when the skin is dry and the limb can be easily gripped without slipping. Performed slowly, safely and with minimal effort, this stretching technique is easy to apply, although it might require a different working posture than the one you are used to. Not only does traction enhance the sensation of deep tissue massage, therapeutically it can significantly improve range of movement in a joint. For this reason it should not be used on clients with joint laxity—those who are hypermobile, have had dislocations or who have unstable joints. You should also avoid using traction on clients with fragile skin because it localizes the stretch in tissues around a joint, including the skin.

One of the best places to practice traction is on the back of the armpit, over the latissimus dorsi, teres major and teres minor muscles. This is often an area much neglected by massage. Here you can traction the glenohumeral joint of the shoulder to stretch many of the associated muscles, which is particularly useful if clients regularly use these muscles as part of a sport or hobby (such as rock climbing or rowing); if they have been using crutches (which requires adduction of the glenohumeral joint); or if tissues have been shortened following surgery in which the arm has been deliberately but temporarily immobilized in an adducted position.

Tractioning the Glenohumeral Joint in Prone

This technique is ideal for improving joint range, which is particularly useful for clients who have limited abduction. Although we have chosen to illustrate the technique with the shoulder abducted to 90 degrees, you can start tractioning at *any* degree of abduction, providing that you are able to get a hold of the elbow in a comfortable manner.

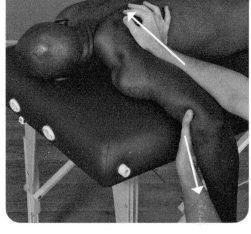

➤ See page 164 for complete instructions on using traction on the glenohumeral joint.

1. With your client prone, carefully abduct his shoulder to around 90 degrees or less.

2. Kneeling down if necessary, place one hand against the back of the client's armpit and use the other to support his elbow.

3. Keeping your own elbow extended, gently press into the back of the armpit while simultaneously tractioning the glenohumeral joint with your other hand. Avoid pressure into the armpit itself, where there are important neural, vascular and lymphatic structures.

TIP Avoid gripping the elbow too tightly. Very little force is required to traction the shoulder in this way. Remember that you are trying to distract the glenohumeral joint, not the elbow joint.

Two Modifications for Tractioning the Glenohumeral Joint in Prone

There are two ways to modify this technique to increase the stretch in the tissues you are working; with each of these, the client is likely to sense an increase in pressure.

First, you can add a small amount of oil to the back of the armpit and then apply the stretch and traction through a facecloth or small towel. Continue to traction the shoulder in the same way, supporting the elbow. Notice that just as the sensation of pressure increased when you applied a transverse stretch to the erector spinae through a cloth (p. 93), so it does here. You can increase this sensation even more should you want to: Instead of keeping your palm flat against the back of the armpit, rotate your palm so that you take up the slack in the underlying skin. Notice that after applying a small amount of oil, you can press through the cloth to get a better grip on the skin and can really stretch the tissues on the back of the armpit.

To further facilitate abduction and stretch in latissimus dorsi, teres major and teres minor muscles, you can passively move the shoulder joint *while tractioning*. Keeping your palm pressed against the tissue of the armpit, simply increase the degree of abduction you are using as you continue to traction the joint. With your palm on the back of the armpit, as usual, direct your stretch inferiorly as you use your other hand to abduct the client's shoulder.

Note that you can easily incorporate this posterior shoulder stretch into an oil massage, using the palm with which you will press to stroke down the client's triceps and up and onto the back of the shoulder.

Table 4.1 shows situations in which you can incorporate tractioning into a deep tissue massage and the chapters in which these situations are discussed.

Table 4.1   Situations in Which Traction Is Useful

	POSITION		
Chapter	Three-quarter lying	Supine	Prone
5	Stretching Latissimus Dorsi	Fisting Pectorals	—
6	—	—	
7	Applying Pressure to Latissimus Dorsi	Using Your Forearm on Triceps Fisting Triceps Fist Wrist Extensors	Working the Posterior Shoulder Tractioning the Glenohumeral Joint Using Your Forearm on Wrist Extensors

Safety Guidelines for Tractioning

Providing you avoid pressure into the armpit itself, tractioning is a safe and effective technique, but it is not suitable for all clients. Traction should not be used on clients who are hypermobile or who have been diagnosed with having a hypermobile syndrome. Although the technique can be used on other parts of the body, avoid applying it to previously dislocated joints or those likely to dislocate (e.g., if a client tells you he has a joint instability). Use traction with medical advice when treating clients with known inflammatory joint conditions, such as rheumatoid arthritis, because this could result in an aggravation of the condition. Traction is not possible to perform on some joints of clients with ankylosing spondylitis or when joints have been fused. This technique also stretches the tissues around a joint, including the skin, so it should be avoided when treating clients with fragile skin. The use of gentle traction is a safe and comfortable adjunct to deep tissue massage for most clients, but if you have doubts it is appropriate for a particular client, consult his or her medical practitioner.

Advantages, Disadvantages and Uses of Tractioning

After practicing how to traction a joint, tick those statements with which you agree in the following three lists:

Advantages

- Tractioning is ideal for improving range of movement in a restricted joint.
- It helps to localize a stretch to a particular area of tissue.
- It is useful when the use of oil is not appropriate or might be problematic.
- It is easy to apply.
- It requires little effort on behalf of the therapist.
- It enhances the sensation of deep tissue massage.
- Tractioning is easily modified to increase the sensation of the stretch.

Disadvantages

- It takes practice to link tractioning into your massage.
- Traction needs to be used selectively; it is not appropriate for all clients.
- It often requires therapists to adopt a different working position to safeguard their posture.

Situations When Tractioning Is Indicated

- When you need to improve range of movement in a restricted joint
- When treating a muscle or area of tissue you have identified as being tight or shortened (usually used when you need to stretch a localized area of tissue)
- When treating a client who requires or values the sensation of exceptionally deep tissue massage

Dry Stretching for the Piriformis Muscle

Let's complete this section on dry stretching by focusing on a specific muscle. Unless our clients are actively engaged in sporting activity, they are unlikely to have a particularly tight gluteus maximus muscle, especially if they are in seated occupations, in which this muscle remains lengthened and weak. However, the gluteus minimus and gluteus medius muscles might be shortened, as might the piriformis. The piriformis muscle is believed to be particularly problematic in manual therapy because of its close proximity to the sciatic nerve. Theoretically, tension in this muscle can press on the nerve, leading to piriformis syndrome. Untreated, the biomechanics of the hip are altered and muscular imbalance ensues. Many therapists are thus keen to learn techniques to allow them to stretch this muscle. One of the best ways is with deep tissue dry stretching.

Using Dry Stretching on the Piriformis Muscle

With your client positioned in the prone position, thoroughly warm the buttocks using your regular massage techniques.

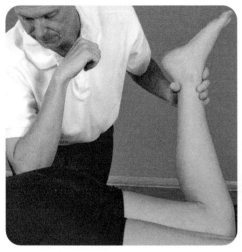 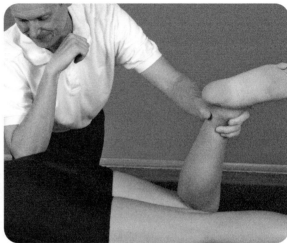

➤ See page 145 for complete instructions on accessing the piriformis muscle.

1. Carefully locate the piriformis muscle. On most clients this will be tender when deep pressure is applied, especially if it is tight.

2. Replace the towel and relocate the muscle. On our photos we have left the towel off so you can easily identify the position in which you need to apply pressure—in the very centre of the buttock.

TIP Working through a towel will get a better stretch on this muscle because you are not at risk of slipping.

3. Lean onto the client using your elbow to 'lock' the piriformis muscle, taking care to support your own back. If the client reports pain, tingling or numbness, use less pressure.

4. With your other hand, hold the client's ankle and slowly rotate the hip joint back and forth *while maintaining pressure with your elbow*. Notice where the client reports the sensation of stretch, and repeat these movements for a few minutes only.

5. Remove the towel and soothe the area.

6. Repeat if necessary, but avoid overworking this area.

Safety Guidelines for Dry Stretching Piriformis

Having thoroughly warmed the area first, always work cautiously, avoiding too much pressure too early. If pressure elicits pain, numbness or tingling in the lower limbs, stop because this indicates you are compressing the sciatic nerve. Always avoid the no-pain-no-gain approach.

Advantages, Disadvantages and Uses of Piriformis Stretching

After practicing stretching the piriformis, tick those statements with which you agree in the following three lists:

Advantages

- Dry stretching is reportedly very effective for stretching the piriformis muscle and thus overcoming problems associated with a tight piriformis.
- The stretch is relatively easy to apply.

Disadvantages

- Because the piriformis lies close to the sciatic nerve, extra caution is needed when performing this technique.
- Not all clients appreciate receiving elbow pressure to the buttock region.

Situations When Dry Stretching to Piriformis Is Indicated

- When you have identified this muscle to be tight and contributing to muscle imbalance in your client
- When a client suffers from piriformis syndrome—a condition in which the piriformis muscle impinges the sciatic nerve (apply stretch with extra caution in this situation)

'With Oil' Stretching

Now let's look at applying stretching techniques with oil, working directly on the skin. In each of the examples described you will see how the elements of tractioning and joint movement may be combined to further enhance the stretch and sensations of pressure. To begin, we'll consider how stretch naturally occurs during the application of compressive techniques. Take a look at this photo of the adductor muscles being treated in supine.

Would you agree that during this compressive effleurage, the fact that the therapist has considerable leverage with respect to the muscles being treated means that these tissues are likely to be stretched during the application of the stroke? In this particular example, the therapist is pushing the skin and fascia proximally, working away from the knee, towards the hip. Would you say that by using less oil there is likely to be more drag against the skin, and the tissues are likely to be stretched even more? Although our intention might be to compress muscles, whenever we work this way stretch occurs. See chapters 6 and 7 for similar examples (in chapter 6, see p. 109, Using Your Forearms on Adductors; p. 126, Using Your Forearm on the Quadriceps; p. 136, Using Your Forearm

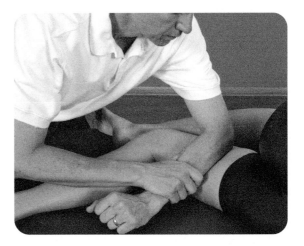

on the Calf; and p. 142, Using Your Forearms on Hamstrings; in chapter 7, see p. 154, Using Your Forearm on Triceps; and p. 165, Using Your Forearm on Wrist Extensors).

In each of these examples a broad area of the muscle and associated fascia is being stretched because the forearm is being used. Stretch also occurs where the stroke being used is narrow, such as when using the elbow (see p. 110, Using Your Elbows on Adductors; p. 113, Using Your Elbow on the Medial Calf; p. 128, Using Your Elbow on the Quadriceps; and p. 132, Applying Your Elbow to Tibialis Anterior). One of the reasons these narrow, stripping-type techniques feel so intense is that they both compress *and* stretch tissues simultaneously.

So, if your intention is to incorporate stretching techniques with oil, you could start simply by positioning yourself to apply some of the compressive techniques just mentioned and, using less oil, intend to stretch tissues as you apply the compressive strokes.

TIP   When you intend to stretch muscles during massage, the effect is quite different from when you intend to compress them. When your intention is to compress tissues, you ask yourself such questions as, 'How can I employ more or less pressure?' and 'What is the effect of adding more pressure in this way?' Once you start to try and stretch tissues, you notice that the *direction* of your strokes is paramount. You will notice that moving in one direction increases the stretch, whereas working in another reduces it.

See table 4.2 for useful examples of practicing stretching with oil, without necessarily adding joint movement, and the chapters to find these examples in. If you use this table to help you choose areas on which to practice the application of oil stretching, choose the forearm treatments first and, once competent, progress to treatments using your fist and then your elbow.

Table 4.2   Situations in Which Naturally Occurring Stretch Can Be Enhanced With Oil

	POSITION		
Chapter	**Three-quarter lying**	**Supine**	**Prone**
5	Using Your Forearm on Upper Trapezius	—	—
6	Using Your Forearms on Adductors Using Your Elbows on Adductors Using Your Fists on Adductors Fisting the Medial Calf Using Your Elbow on the Medial Calf	Using Your Forearm on the Quadriceps Using Your Elbow on the Quadriceps Using Your Forearm on the Adductors Applying Your Elbow to Tibialis Anterior	Using Your Forearm on the Calf Using Your Elbow on the Calf Fisting the Calf Fisting the Calf With Dorsiflexion Using Your Forearm to Apply Soft Tissue Release Using Your Forearms on Hamstrings Using Your Elbows on Hamstrings
7	—	Using Your Forearm on Triceps Fisting Triceps Fisting Biceps Fist Wrist Extensors	Using Your Forearm on Wrist Extensors

Stretching With Oil Plus a Passive Joint Movement

To further enhance a stretch you can move the joint associated with the muscles on which you are working. You can do this passively or ask the client to move the joint. Both methods are described here.

A good way to explore the technique of stretch and joint movement is treating the calf with the client prone. The advantage of this scenario is that you can perform the stretch passively or ask the client to perform the stretch.

Using Stretching With Oil Plus a Passive Joint Movement

The technique of stretching with oil and passive joint movement is described here using the calf as an example. Following the steps, you should easily be able to adapt this technique to most limb joints.

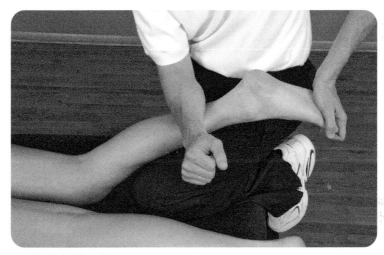

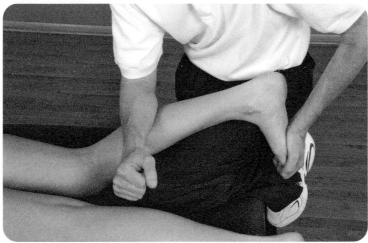

➤ See page 140 for complete instructions on using your forearm to apply soft tissue release to the calves.

1. Passively shorten the muscle. In the case of the calf, this means either flexing the knee or plantar flexing the ankle, or both. In the photo, the therapist has flexed the client's knee but left the client's ankle in a neutral position (that is, neither overly plantar flexed nor dorsiflexed).

2. Starting at the distal end of the muscle, use a little oil to apply a compressive effleurage type stroke, working proximally. In this case you are working from the ankle towards the knee, avoiding pressure into the popliteal space at the back of the knee.

TIP The key here is to maintain pressure in the effleurage stroke during movement of the joint. If you are passively stretching the muscles, this requires you to be ambidextrous, applying forearm effleurage with one arm while dorsiflexing the client's ankle with the other.

3. Repeat this stroke, but this time stretch the muscle on which you are working. In the case of the calf, this means dorsiflexing the ankle. You can do this passively or ask your client to do it.

TIP Active dorsiflexion of the ankle by the client results in a greater relaxation in ankle plantar flexors (such as the gastrocnemius and soleus) as the client engages the tibialis anterior, the antagonist to these muscles. Remember that muscles work in pairs, so contracting one muscle produces relaxation in its opposite. However, the disadvantage of repeated use of active movements is that this could fatigue the muscles being contracted—in this example, the tibialis anterior muscle.

4. Repeat the stroke three or four times, with dorsiflexion.

Notice this is particularly effective at treating the middle and lateral aspects of the calf because you can more easily access these areas with your effleurage stroke. Notice too that you cannot easily traction this particular joint. Compare the previous two photos with the following photo to see how the technique can easily be applied to the forearm, where it is useful in increasing wrist flexion. When used on the forearm it is easier to also traction the joint by gently pulling on the wrist as you also passively flex it. Notice that to apply the technique to the wrist you must position your client so that this joint can be flexed; to do this, his hand needs to be resting over the end of the treatment couch.

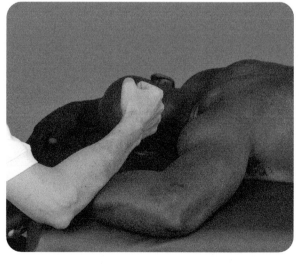

➤ See page 165 for more information on this form of deep tissue stretching.

Stretching With Oil Plus an Active Joint Movement

In some situations, movement of the joint is best performed by the client, enabling the therapist to focus on facilitating the stretch. Good examples are when treating the ilio-tibial band on the lateral side of the thigh, and when treating the hamstrings in supine. In both cases the therapist has less leverage than in the examples previously described, so he or she has slightly less compressive force at disposal; plus, applying the stretch while *also* moving the associated joint would be difficult.

Stretching the ITB With Oil Plus Joint Movement

Follow these steps to safely stretch the ITB.

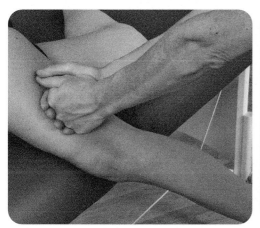 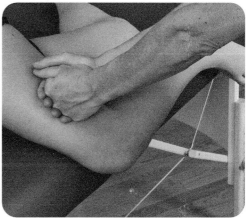

➤ See page 117 for complete instructions on applying soft tissue release to the ITB.

1. Position your client in three-quarter lying so that her knee rests on the edge of the treatment couch.

TIP If this is uncomfortable, place a folded towel or bath sponge beneath her knee.

2. With loosely cupped fists and trying to keep your elbows extended, apply pressure to the distal end of the vastus lateralis muscle, just superior to the knee joint. Take care not to press too deeply into the lateral epicondyle of the femur in this region.

3. Using a little oil, slowly fist up the iliotibial band as your client *slowly* flexes and extends her knee.

TIP Knowing where to stand to avoid being kicked by a client's moving foot requires practice. Stretching the ITB with oil plus joint movement is a tricky technique on clients with long legs!

4. Repeat three or four times.

Stretching in this way is particularly helpful for targeting localized areas of tension around a joint. Stretching the iliotibial band is reported to be helpful in treating conditions such as runner's knee (iliotibial band friction syndrome), in which tension in the lateral retinaculum of the knee might be a contributing factor. The value of active stretching is the client is in control at all times over the severity of the stretch. If clients feel the stretch is too strong, they simply stop moving that limb. Alternatively, the therapist could apply less pressure to the stretch, and together the client and therapist can work up to a tolerable level in order to meet the treatment outcomes. The downsides to active stretching are that not all clients want to take part in treatment in this way, and that to move a joint the client must be in a position in which this is possible.

Compare the technique just described to the technique described on page 121 (Using Your Forearm on Hamstrings) for treating the hamstrings in supine. Note that when treating the hamstrings in this way you can ask your client to straighten his leg as you use your forearm to effleurage from just inferior to the knee joint to the hip. As the client straightens his leg, the sensation of stretch will increase. You cannot, however, use this technique everywhere. Look at the use of forearms and elbows to the quadriceps in supine (pp. 126 and 128, Using Your Forearm on the Quadriceps and Using Your Elbow on the Quadriceps). In these situations neither you nor the client can increase the stretch because to do so you would need to flex the knee, which you cannot do in a supine position.

See table 4.3 for examples of situations in which to use stretching with oil plus joint movement, and the chapters to find them in.

Adding Traction

In some places you can stretch tissues further by combining traction with your movement of the joint. This is easier than it sounds and works best on the upper limb. Of all the techniques described in this chapter, this is the most advanced because it requires you to perform several movements at once. However, you might already be doing this instinctively. Turn to page 165 (Using Your Forearm on Wrist Extensors), where you can see the wrist extensors being treated. Here you were learning to combine flexion of the wrist with deep stretching massage to the wrist extensor muscles. Can you see how you could also gently traction the wrist as you do this, pulling the wrist towards you with one hand as you apply deep effleurage away from you with your other forearm?

See table 4.4 for examples of situations in which this very advanced technique might be used.

Safety Guidelines for 'With Oil' Stretching

Avoid pressing too deeply over bony points, such as the lateral epicondyles of the femur when treating the iliotibial band. Remember that when a client actively moves a joint, this is beneficial for reducing tone in the muscle being stretched, but if he or she moves the joint too many times the muscle being contracted will fatigue. Do not use deep tissue stretching on clients with fragile skin or on clients who are hypermobile or who have hypermobility syndromes. Avoid deep tissue stretching when its use will increase

Table 4.3 Situations in Which (Active or Passive) Joint Movement Is Useful

	POSITION		
Chapter	Three-quarter lying	Supine	Prone
5	—	Fisting Trapezius Fisting Pectorals	—
6	Applying Soft Tissue Release to the ITB	Using Your Forearm on Hamstrings Fisting Hamstrings	Using Your Forearm on the Calf Using Your Elbow on the Calf Fisting the Calf Using Your Forearm to Apply Soft Tissue Release Using Your Forearms on Hamstrings Using Your Elbows on Hamstrings
7	Applying Pressure to Latissimus Dorsi	Using Your Forearm on Triceps Fisting Biceps	Working the Posterior Shoulder Using Your Forearm on Wrist Extensors

Table 4.4 Situations in Which Adding Traction Is Useful

	POSITION		
Chapter	Three-quarter lying	Supine	Prone
5	Stretching Latissimus Dorsi	Fisting Trapezius Fisting Pectorals	—
6	—	—	—
7	Applying Pressure to Latissimus Dorsi	Using Your Forearm on Triceps Fisting Triceps Fisting Biceps	Working the Posterior Shoulder Tractioning the Glenohumeral Joint Using Your Forearm on Wrist Extensors

mobility in an unstable joint. If you intend to incorporate tractioning with oil stretching, be sure to read the safety guidelines for this technique on page 64.

Advantages, Disadvantages and Uses of Stretching with Oil

After practicing stretching with oil, tick those statements with which you agree in the following three lists:

Advantages

- Stretching with oil is ideal for improving range of movement in a restricted joint.
- It helps localize a stretch to a particular area of tissue.
- It requires little effort from the therapist once the technique has been mastered.
- It enhances the sensation of deep tissue massage.

Disadvantages

- The client needs to be positioned in such a way that movement of the joint is possible.
- The technique needs to be used selectively and is not appropriate for all clients.
- The technique takes time to learn and master, especially when a joint is moved passively and the therapist is required to be ambidextrous.

Situations When 'With Oil' Stretching Is Indicated

- When you need to improve range of movement in a restricted joint
- When treating a muscle or area of tissue you have identified as being tight, or shortened
- When treating a client who requires the sensation of exceptionally deep tissue massage
- When you wish to apply deep tissue massage but do not have adequate leverage for pure compressive techniques
- When the use of stretching might be more effective than massage alone

Closing Remarks

Now you have learned stretching techniques both with and without oil and can use these along with compressive techniques to deliver deep tissue massage. In the next chapters you will learn to use these techniques for treating different parts of the body, starting with the trunk.

Quick Questions

1. When dry stretching, how can you enhance the sensation of deep pressure?
2. For which clients is tractioning not appropriate?
3. What is the advantage of asking a client to actively move a joint while you apply stretch with oil?
4. When treating the wrist extensors, why do you position the client with his or her wrist off the end of the treatment couch?
5. In which situations is it difficult to move joints passively?

PART III

Applying Deep Tissue Massage

Here we come to the nuts and bolts of deep tissue massage. The three chapters in this part of the book provide detailed information about the application of deep tissue techniques to the trunk (chapter 5), lower limbs (chapter 6) and upper limbs (chapter 7). Within each chapter, techniques have been grouped according to the position in which the client receives treatment: three-quarter lying, supine or prone, and seated when applicable. We start with the three-quarter-lying position because many readers will not have used this position before. This part of the book gives you a structure with which to practice the techniques (the order in which the photographs are presented is not intended to form a routine). For information on how to put together a deep tissue massage routine in each of these positions, see chapter 8.

Techniques shown in this section of the book include both compression and stretch; tools are used when appropriate. Most of the techniques included here are unlikely to have been covered during your initial massage training course, unless this course contained a postcourse advanced module. Enjoy practicing with these deep tissue methods, all of which are safe and effective. As you know, different clients have different preferences, and it would be useful if you could make time to receive treatment yourself so that you have a greater understanding of how each technique feels to receive in each of the three positions. Answering the questions at the end of each chapter will help consolidate your knowledge and prepare you to incorporate your new skills into a routine of your choice.

A Note on the Three-Quarter-Lying Position

This is a position similar to the recovery position in first aid. In the recovery position, a person is rolled from a side-lying position almost onto the abdomen, with their uppermost leg slightly flexed at the hip and knee. If you try to treat the client in the recovery position, you might find that you cannot get leverage on certain muscles as effectively as when the client is in the three-quarter-lying position. Whenever you are practicing techniques that call for clients to be placed in the three-quarter-lying position, it is likely that you will need to ask them to lie on their side first. You can then help them adjust their neck and limbs to suit the treatment you are about to provide. Most clients quickly become familiar with this position and know how to get into it when asked. As an alternative, you can position your clients on their side, but the disadvantage to this is that most clients tense their muscles once you start massaging them because this position requires them to stay balanced on their iliac crest and greater trochanter.

Deep Tissue Massage for the Trunk

In this chapter you will find 30 photographs and instructions for applying deep tissue massage to all major muscles of the trunk, including the trapezius, levator scapulae, rhomboids, erector spinae, pectorals, quadratus lumborum and latissimus dorsi (see table 5.1). Techniques are grouped according to the positions in which they are usefully applied: three-quarter lying, supine, prone and seated. You will also find tips to help you apply these techniques.

Table 5.1   Muscles Targeted by Deep Tissue Massage Techniques Included in This Chapter

Muscle	POSITION			
	Three-quarter lying	Supine	Prone	Seated
Upper trapezius	✓	✓	✓	✓
Middle/lower trapezius	—	With ball	✓	—
Levator scapulae	✓	With ball	✓	✓
Rhomboids	—	With ball	✓	—
Latissimus dorsi	✓	—	—	—
Quadratus lumborum	✓	—	—	—
Erector spinae	—	—	✓	✓
Pectorals	—	✓	—	—
Occipital muscles	—	✓	✓	—

We will start with three-quarter lying, a position you might not have used before. Notice that in each of these techniques for the trunk, the side of the body to be treated is the side uppermost to the therapist. This is not always the case with three-quarter lying massage. Compare the following three-quarter lying techniques with those for the adductors (p. 109) in which the side being treated is the side against the couch.

Using Your Forearm on Upper Trapezius

Step 1: Position your client so you have access to the neck and upper fibers of the trapezius. This is a technique that requires you to sit or to kneel in order to prevent excessive unsupported flexion of your own spine.

TIP Many clients prefer to have some form of support beneath the head, such as a pillow or small folded towel. However, if possible, try to keep the neck in either a neutral position or a position slightly flexed *away* from you. Having the neck slightly flexed means you are working through lengthened rather than shortened fibers, and the technique will feel more powerful.

Step 2: Apply oil to your forearm and, keeping your wrist loose, gently sweep your forearm from the occiput all the way down the neck, gliding gently over the shoulder. Practice a few times, applying deeper pressure as you sweep over the belly of the upper fibers of the trapezius but applying gentler pressure over bony areas such as the transverse and spinous processes of the cervical vertebrae, the shoulder and the spine of the scapula.

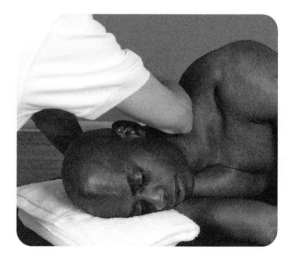

TIP Aim to apply your pressure perpendicular to the muscle. If this feels awkward, change your own body position and try again.

Advantages   This is a great technique for getting into the upper fibers of the trapezius, especially useful when treating clients with short necks. ■ It might easily be linked to the next technique for treating the levator scapulae, and when treating the deltoid in this position (see p. 151). ■ Using this same position to apply compression only, this might be used as a 'dry' technique (through clothing without oil).

Disadvantage   The therapist will definitely need to sit or kneel to apply this technique.

Using Your Elbow on Levator Scapulae

Step 1: Position your client as for the treatment of the upper fibers of trapezius, lengthening these fibers slightly, if possible.

Step 2: Locate the levator scapulae where it inserts onto the superior angle of the scapula. Move so that you are not on the bone, and apply gentle but firm pressure using your elbow. The muscle is easily accessed in this position, so take care not to go too deep too soon. Again, aim to apply your pressure perpendicular to the tissue being treated and practice from different seated (or kneeling) positions.

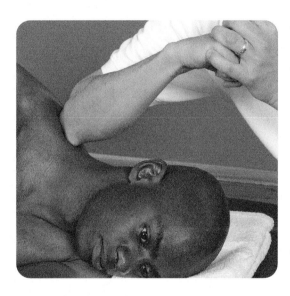

TIP For clients who require greater pressure, simply reinforce your hand and use your body weight to gently lean into the point of pressure.

Advantage This is a very effective way to access the levator scapulae.

Disadvantages Because the levator scapulae (a muscle in which many clients feel tension) is easily accessed in this position, the technique might be too powerful for some clients. ■ The therapist will definitely need to sit or to kneel to apply this technique.

Stretching Latissimus Dorsi

Step 1: Apply a small amount of oil to your palm and gently abduct the client's uppermost arm.

Step 2: Starting from the armpit, apply firm pressure and gently glide down the latissimus dorsi muscle, taking care as you press over the ribs. If possible, glide all the way to the iliac crest.

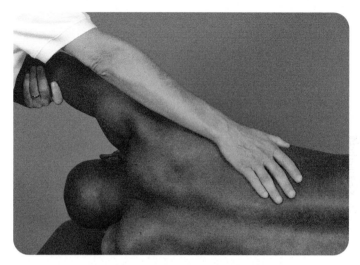

CLIENT TALK

Combined with work to the teres muscles (see chapter 7), I regularly used this stretch to latissimus dorsi on a client who had been forced to use crutches because of a fractured ankle. The muscles that adducted his humerus were exceptionally tight, and he gained much relief from being stretched in this position. Unable to receive treatment prone or supine because of the pressure this would place on his ankle, he received all his treatment in the three-quarter-lying position.

Advantages   This technique helps to both compress and stretch the latissimus dorsi, so it is potentially beneficial for clients who use this muscle as part of their sport (e.g., rock climbers or rowers) or for clients who have been using crutches when humeral adduction is required. ■ The technique can be modified to include the triceps muscle, starting here and working along the triceps, over the back of the armpit and into the latissimus dorsi.

Disadvantages   It is difficult to keep female clients adequately towel draped when performing this movement because it is best applied against the skin when the client is not wearing underwear. ■ This technique can be tiring to perform on large clients with heavy arms or on tall clients when it is not possible to glide all the way to the iliac crest.

Forearm Sweep

Step 1: In three-quarter-lying position, your client has his uppermost arm above his head, thus opening the thorax and lumbar areas for treatment.

Step 2: Starting at the client's waist with both of your elbows together, sweep your forearms apart gently, gliding one forearm over the ribs and the other down towards the iliac crest. To vary the technique, work a much smaller area, leaning in towards the client so that you stretch and compress the quadratus lumborum in this position. Always take care to avoid any deep pressure around the 12th rib and the kidney area.

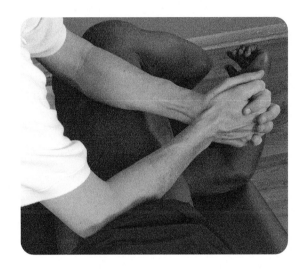

Advantages This technique can help link trunk work to the treatment of the shoulder or gluteals in three-quarter lying. ▪ Some clients love the sensation of being 'opened out' in this position, which not only helps to lengthen the fibers of the quadratus lumborum but also the uppermost ribs and muscles of the armpit.

Disadvantages Some clients dislike the sensation of forearms against their ribs. ▪ It might be difficult to adequately towel drape female clients to receive this treatment, which is best performed against skin with the client's underwear removed.

Using Your Forearm on Quadratus Lumborum

Step 1: In three-quarter-lying position, your client has his uppermost arm above his head, as for the previous technique.

Step 2: Using one forearm only this time, gently press into the tissues of the lumbar area, sweeping down towards the iliac crest. Pressure should be light over the ribs and kidney area, and deeper as you approach the iliac crest, but easing off over the crest itself.

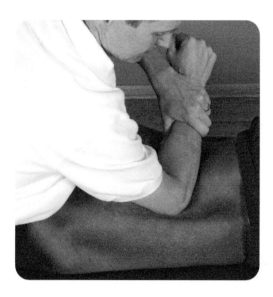

TIP For even better access to this area, place a small folded towel or small diameter bolster beneath the client's waist, thus eliciting slight lateral flexion away from the uppermost side.

Advantages   This is a great technique to help access a tight quadratus lumborum muscle or for chronically tight lumbar extensors. ▪ The client may alter the position of the upper arm to change the degree of stretch experienced; greatest stretch is achieved with the arm above the head. ▪ This technique is easily linked to the next, even deeper, technique.

Disadvantage   Therapists need to fully support themselves when applying this technique, perhaps by resting on the couch.

Using Your Elbow on Quadratus Lumborum

Step 1: Position your client either with arms above the head, as in the previous two techniques, or in front of the body, as shown in the photo.

Step 2: Using your elbow, apply firm but gentle pressure into the lumbar area. Focus your pressure on the lower inner quadrant of quadratus lumborum, avoiding the lowest ribs and the kidney area.

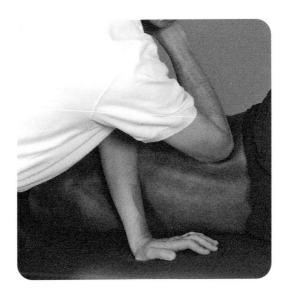

Advantage This is a powerful technique on chronically tight lumbar extensor muscles.

Disadvantage It can take time to locate the trigger points in quadratus lumborum because this is a very deep muscle covering a relatively small area.

TIP Think of quadratus lumborum as a lawn in which you need to find one or two hidden moleholes. Instead of working randomly over the muscle, imagine mowing that lawn with an old-fashioned mower, moving in lines up and down and then side to side, each time gently applying pressure with your elbow. Sooner or later you will discover the spot that the client feels is most beneficial for deep pressure.

Here we present tips on applying some well-known techniques more deeply, plus some ideas for using tools.

Fisting Trapezius

Step 1: Massage the upper trapezius as you would normally in supine.

Step 2: Instead of keeping the head in a neutral position, gently flex it away from you as you use your fist to stroke from the base of the skull to the shoulder. Keep your fixed hand against the client's head. This creates a slight stretch in the upper fibers of trapezius, made more intense with the application of massage.

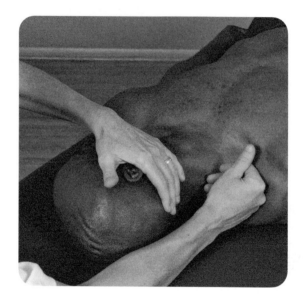

Advantage   This is an easy technique to incorporate into a regular routine for the upper trapezius muscle.

Using a Tool on Trapezius

Step 1: Having thoroughly warmed the area first, locate a trigger spot in the upper fibers of trapezius and carefully position a massage tool there.

Step 2: Using the tool, apply gentle but firm pressure, requesting feedback from your client. Hold the tool in place for around 30 seconds, and then gently ease off your pressure and soothe the area.

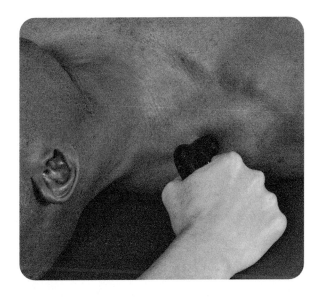

TIP Once you have applied the pressure, gently tap the client's opposite shoulder as you maintain pressure with the tool. This sends a different sensory message and serves as a form of distraction to any discomfort the client feels from the deep pressure.

Advantage   This is a great technique for saving therapists' thumbs. Most clients cannot feel the difference between the use of a massage tool and the therapist's thumb.

Disadvantage   If you have not used a massage tool before, this treatment will take practice.

Using a Tennis Ball

Step 1: Using a tennis ball, help your client locate trigger points in the trapezius, rhomboids and even levator scapulae muscles. These are found in the fleshy parts of the muscle.

Step 2: Once the spot is located and the ball is in place, time your client as he rests in this position on the ball for no more than 45 seconds. The sensation he feels should be one commonly known by massage therapists as 'grateful pain'. Remove the ball and locate another spot.

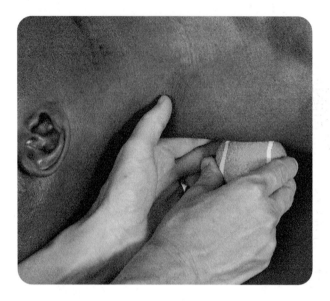

Advantage   This technique works well for teaching clients to treat their own trigger spots.

Disadvantage   Remember that the client has his body weight resting on the ball, focusing pressure to one particular spot, so take care to ensure the ball does not rest on a bony structure such as the spine or scapulae.

Stretching Pectorals

Step 1: This simple stretch is often used at the start of a treatment in supine, but it can be made more powerful and form part of a deep tissue routine by placing a rolled-up towel or bolster longitudinally down the length of the client's thoracic spine, taking care to also support the head.

Step 2: With the towel or bolster in place, gently lean onto your client's shoulders, pressing them to the couch and stretching the pectorals.

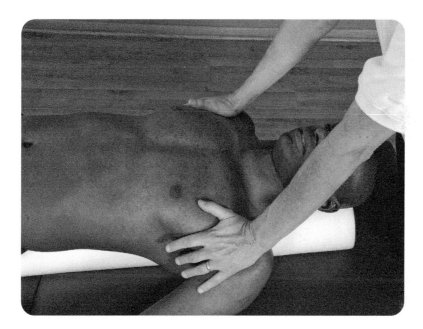

CLIENT TALK

This pectoral stretch in supine was used in the treatment of a female client who spent many hours daily sitting at a computer. Each session we would start her treatment with me simply resting on her shoulders, gently stretching the pectorals, which had become short and tight.

Advantage   This is an extremely powerful stretch for clients with kyphotic postures, in which the pectoral muscles are shortened.

TIP If pressure against the anterior of the shoulder is uncomfortable for your client, try pressing through a bath sponge.

Applying Digital Pressure to Pectorals

Step 1: Using just the pads of your fingers, locate the coracoid process of the scapula.

Step 2: Glide your fingers repeatedly, working from the sternum to the coracoid, trying not to press into the ribs. Little pressure is needed in this area, but reinforce your hands, if necessary.

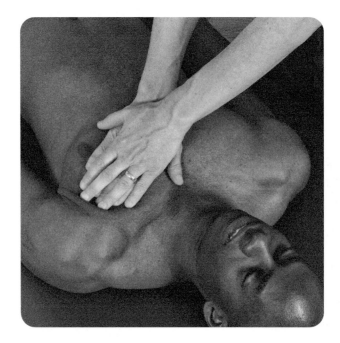

Advantage   This is a good alternative technique for the treatment of tight pectoral muscles.

Disadvantages   This technique might not be appropriate for all female clients, especially those with large breasts, because their breasts might intrude on the treatment area. ■ The coracoid area is often very sore in clients with kyphotic postures and in cases in which the pectoralis minor, biceps brachii and coracobrachialis muscles are tight because these all insert into this process.

Fisting Pectorals

Step 1: Hold your client's arm away from the treatment couch, in shoulder flexion.

Step 2: Using oil, gently glide your fist from the insertion of pectoralis major on the humerus towards the sternum. Obviously, on male clients the treatable area is larger. Notice what happens if you lower your client's arm to the couch while applying the stroke. You should find that the pressure intensifies as the fibers of pectoralis major start to lengthen in this abducted position.

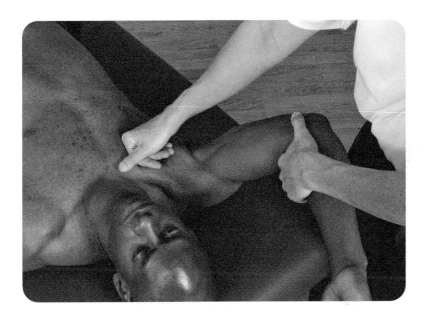

Advantage   This method is useful for applying both compression and stretch with oil to this part of the pectoralis major muscle.

Disadvantages   The technique can be tiring to perform on clients with heavy arms. ■ The technique is not appropriate for all female clients, especially those with large breasts.

Applying Digital Pressure to the Occipital Region

Step 1: While seated, slide your fingers, with or without oil, up the back of the client's neck until you reach the occipital bone at the base of the skull.

Step 2: Gently flex your fingers and apply traction. Allow the client to relax his head in this position. To apply more pressure to one side of the head than to the other, gently tilt the client's head onto the fingers of one of your hands.

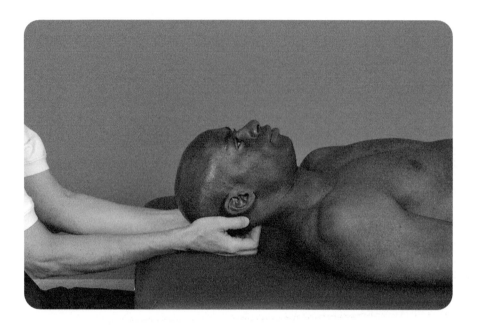

Advantage The insertion of trapezius into the occipital bone is often an area that is sore on clients. Gentle compression and traction of tissues tends to alleviate this discomfort.

Disadvantage Heads are heavy, so performing this technique many times on larger clients can make your finger flexors ache.

Applying Digital Pressure to Cervical Muscles

Step 1: With the client supine, gently flex the head and neck away from the side you wish to work.

Step 2: Using the tips of your fingers, apply gentle pressure to the neck extensor muscles, working along them and requesting feedback from your client. Once you have located areas of tension, either work this area more, using small deep strokes, or as an alternative, ask the client to slowly turn his head towards you, gently pressing into your fingers. Allow him to remain in this position for around 30 seconds; then release and soothe the area.

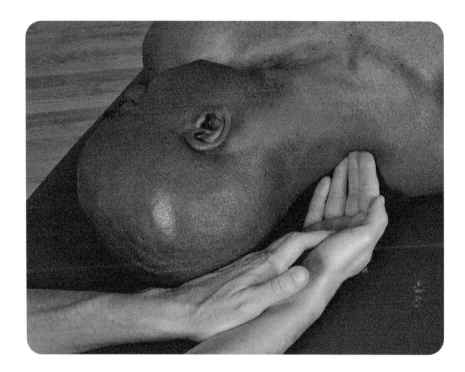

Advantage   This is a useful method of accessing cervical extensor muscles in supine.

Disadvantage   The technique might be uncomfortable for the therapist and should be used selectively to avoid overuse of the therapist's fingers.

Applying Gentle Pressure Beneath the Ribs

Step 1: Locate the rib cage (as shown) and explain to your client that you are going to apply gentle pressure as he exhales. Note that your thumb is used only to locate the ribs in this position but not to apply pressure.

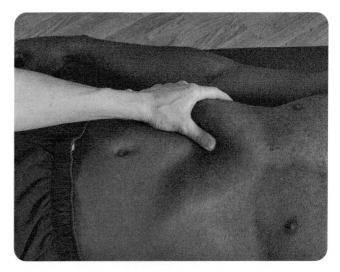

Step 2: Reinforcing your thumb or applying gentle pressure with cupped fingers, ask your client to inhale, and as he breathes out, gently press up and into the diaphragm. It is important that your pressure comes from your reinforcing fingers and not your thumb, the joint of which is compromised in this position.

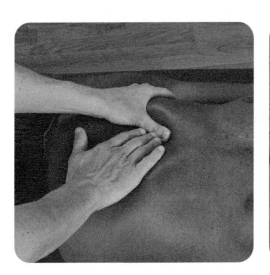 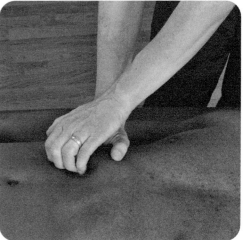

Advantage   This technique can help release tension in the diaphragm and abdomen of some clients.

Disadvantage   Some clients might find the technique too invasive.

These techniques for applying deep tissue massage with the client prone are easily incorporated into a full-body routine.

Transverse Stretching to Erector Spinae

Step 1: Before adding oil, try this gentle transverse stretch to the erector spinae muscles. Locate the spine, and position your palms on the erector spinae muscles farthest from you.

Step 2: Hook the base of your palm into the tissues and firmly press them away from the spine. Work from the upper thoracic area down to the lumbar area and back up again several times. You want to compress and stretch the tissues at the same time. Then move to the other side of the treatment couch to work the opposite erector spinae muscles. Note if any area feels particularly restricted, or if one side of the body seems more tight than the other.

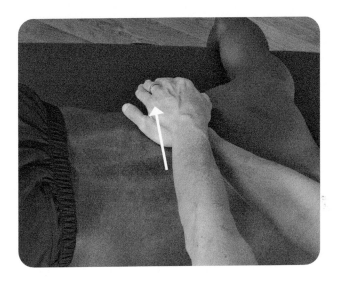

TIP For a really good grip, apply a little oil to the area and perform the technique through a facecloth or small towel.

Advantages This technique loosens the soft tissue and might be used as a dry treatment (without oil). ■ The technique provides a nice alternative to the longitudinal strokes often used in back massage.

Pulling Through Trapezius

Step 1: Using only a little oil, cup the upper fibers of the trapezius on the side of the body farthest from you, using reinforced hands.

Step 2: Pull through these fibers, dragging your fingers through the muscle as you use your body weight to lean back.

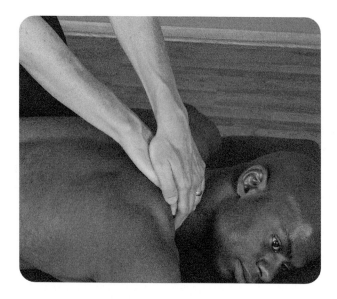

Advantage   An adjunct to petrissage, this technique works the upper fibers of trapezius transversely.

Using Your Forearm on the Lumbar Region

Step 1: Locate the spine and gently rest your forearm over the spinal extensor muscles.

Step 2: Lean into the client as you glide slowly from the lumbar to the thoracic area, taking care to ease up with your pressure as you glide over the ribs.

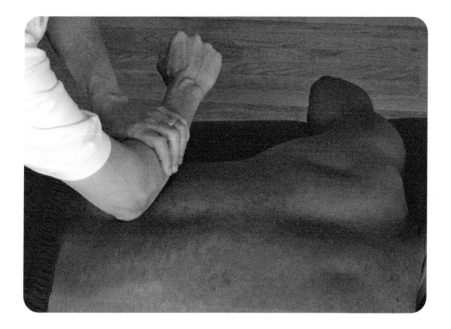

Advantage   This technique is a firm and secure way to apply deep pressure to the erector spinae group.

Disadvantage   Take care to avoid pressing into the spine with the elbow while applying this technique.

Using Your Forearm on Trapezius

Step 1: Locate the medial border of the scapula and the spine. This technique lets you apply deep pressure to the rhomboid muscles, pressing through middle fibers of the trapezius.

Step 2: Lean into the fleshy part of the muscles to compress them. Add oil if you like, and practice gliding your forearm through these muscles while maintaining compression. With care, you can slowly flex your elbow over the areas that require deep work, avoiding pressing into ribs or other bony structures. With practice, you will learn to glide safely between the scapula and the spine, pressing through the upper fibers of the trapezius and into the levator scapulae.

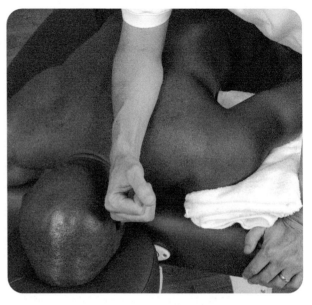

TIP Placing a rolled towel (as in the photo) or thin bolster beneath the shoulder and arm places the upper fibers of the trapezius and rhomboid muscles in a passively shortened position, making them easier to work into. Practice this technique both with and without shoulder support. Can you feel the difference?

CLIENT TALK

I used this technique of shoulder support to treat a female client who had taken up indoor rock climbing as a hobby. She was working out in a gym, aiming to strengthen her rhomboid muscles, and benefited from treatment in this position following training sessions.

Advantages   This is a great method for accessing the rhomboids and working into the upper fibers of the trapezius. ■ Using the shoulder support allows easier access to the levator scapulae and rhomboids minor.

Disadvantage   Clients with exceptionally tight pectorals or anterior deltoid muscle fibers might find the use of a towel uncomfortable.

Using Your Forearm on Trapezius (With Arm Abducted)

Step 1: For an alternative to the previous technique, sit close to the client and place his arm over your thigh, as shown in the photo. This has the same effect for passively shortening the upper fibers of trapezius as using a towel.

Step 2: Lean into the fleshy parts of the muscles, taking care to avoid the spine and scapula. Glide across the fibers using oil, or simply compress the tissues by leaning into them.

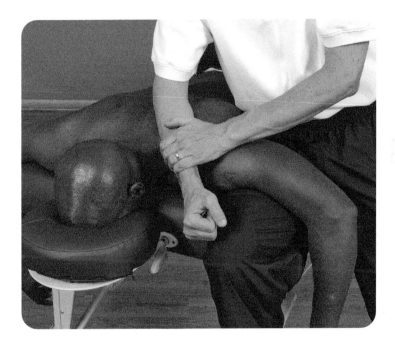

Advantages   This technique is easily combined with massage to the triceps in this same position.   ▪ This position is useful for passive mobilization of the shoulder.   ▪ Passive shortening of the upper fibers of the trapezius allows easier access to the deeper muscles, such as the levator scapulae and rhomboids.

Disadvantage   Some therapists might find the positioning of the client's arm over the thigh inappropriate.

Using Your Elbow on Trapezius

Step 1: For a completely different sensation, try using your forearm from a top-down position. Locate the spine and the medial border of the scapula and position your elbow ready to apply pressure.

Step 2: Once assured that you are on muscle and not bone, slowly but firmly lean into the tissues, taking care to support yourself on the treatment couch to avoid unsupported flexion of your own spine.

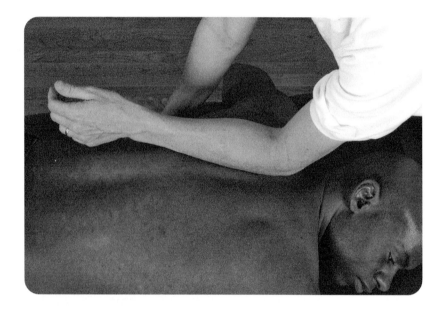

TIP Start with a relatively small degree of elbow flexion. Notice that when you flex your elbow just a few degrees more, the result is a disproportionate degree of pressure experienced by the client.

Advantage   This technique is a good way to access the levator scapulae.

Disadvantage   The leverage that you have as a therapist in this position is considerable, so work with caution.

Applying Digital Pressure to the Neck Muscles

Step 1: Stretch the posterior tissues of the client's neck by applying gentle pressure to the occipital bone at the base of the skull.

Step 2: Using reinforced fingers, work gently into the cervical extensor muscles.

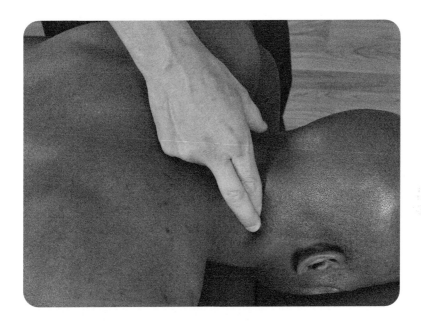

Advantage   Gentle traction aids the application of this technique, which is particularly useful for clients with lordotic necks.

Disadvantage   Overworking these tissues against the cervical vertebrae risks bruising them.

Applying Digital Pressure to the Occipital Region

Step 1: If you are not already using this technique, practice hooking into the occipital bone, the insertion of trapezius and an area of many small cervical muscles.

Step 2: Gently but firmly apply traction, maintaining the position of your fingers.

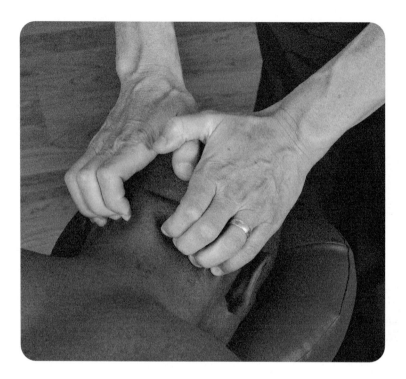

Advantage   This technique provides an additional release to cervical extensor muscles in addition to other techniques you might be using.

Disadvantage   This technique may not provide deep enough pressure for some clients.

Being able to treat clients in a seated position is useful because not all clients are comfortable prone. For example, a client with a painful patella might want a back massage but feels uncomfortable when face down. One of the best ways to position clients is to have them straddle a chair and lean forward with their chest supported on pillows and their feet flat on the floor.

Using Forearms With the Client Seated

Step 1: With your client comfortably seated, perhaps resting forward on a pillow, place your forearm against the upper trapezius.

Step 2: Simply lean towards your client, compressing the tissues in this area. Work over the area, focusing on those places where the client feels most release.

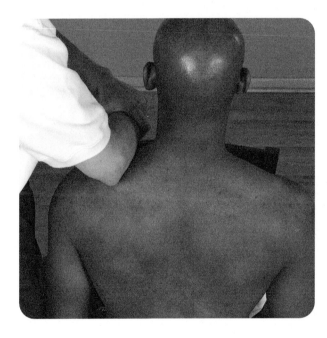

Advantages This technique is useful for compressing the upper fibers of the trapezius when therapists have strong leverage because they can use their body weight. ■ You can use this technique through clothing as a stand-alone compressive technique.

Using Elbows With the Client Seated

Step 1: For even deeper pressure, use your elbow. Start by locating the fleshy part of the muscle, or even the levator scapulae, taking care not to press into the superior angle of the scapulae into which the levator scapulae inserts.

Step 2: Gently lean onto your client until you achieve the degree of pressure required.

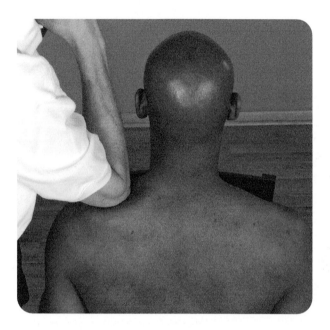

Advantages   This technique allows for more specific compression of tissues. ▪ This is an ideal technique for clients who crave extremely deep pressure in this area, or for whom supine and prone techniques are ineffective.

Disadvantages   Because the therapist can exert considerable leverage in this position, care must be taken in applying the technique. ▪ Pressure as specific as this is not tolerated by all clients.

Treating Erector Spinae With the Client Seated

Step 1: Try this technique for clients with persistently tight extensor muscles. Seat the client on a stool, with chest and arms supported by the treatment couch. Use pillows if necessary for client's comfort.

Step 2: Locate the spine and, using either your forearm or fist, compress the tissues, gliding over them with just a little oil.

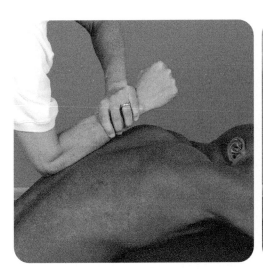 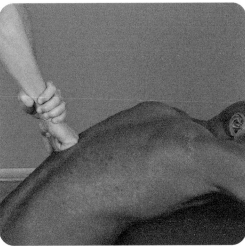

Advantage   This technique provides an alternative approach to the treatment of these muscles, which are usually treated with the client in prone position.

Disadvantages   It might be uncomfortable for some clients to adopt this position. ■ It might be difficult to treat more than just a small section of the erector spinae muscles.

Treating the Lumbar Area With the Client Flexed at the Hip

Step 1: This is a really powerful method of both compressing and stretching the spinal extensor muscles. Position the client so that he is supported on the end of the treatment couch. Place pillows or bolsters beneath his chest for support and comfort, and provide a stool on which he can rest his knees.

Step 2: Working from the lumbar area upwards, lean into the tissues as you gently glide across them. Avoid deep pressure to the lower ribs and kidney area.

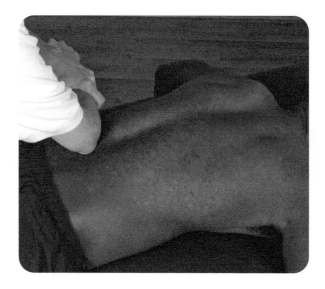

Advantage   This technique is an unusual but alternative method of treating chronically tight spinal extensors.

Disadvantage   This is certainly not a position suitable for all clients to adopt during treatment.

Quick Questions

1. When using your elbow to treat the quadratus lumborum muscle, with your client in a three-quarter-lying position, to which structures should you avoid deep pressure?

2. When treating the upper fibers of the trapezius with a supine client, for how long should you compress tissues using a massage tool?

3. When treating the diaphragm, do you apply your pressure when the client inhales or exhales?

4. When treating the erector spinae muscles transversely with a prone client, what can you do to increase your grip on the tissues?

5. Why might you place a towel beneath a client's shoulder when treating his rhomboids and upper trapezius in prone position?

Deep Tissue Massage for the Lower Limbs

In this chapter you will find photographs and instructions for applying deep tissue massage to the adductors, calves, hamstrings, feet, quadriceps, tibialis anterior and the gluteals (see table 6.1). Also included are techniques for treating the small and much-neglected tensor fascia latae muscle and the iliotibial band. As you know, the iliotibial band is not a muscle, but it is tight in many clients, and many therapists search for

Table 6.1 Muscles Targeted by Deep Tissue Massage Techniques Included in This Chapter

Muscle	POSITION		
	Three-quarter lying	Supine	Prone
Adductors	✓	✓	—
Calf	✓	✓	✓
Achilles	✓	—	—
ITB	✓	✓	—
Buttock	✓	—	✓
TFL	✓	✓	—
Hamstrings	—	✓	✓
Quadriceps	—	✓	—
Tibialis anterior	—	✓	✓
Plantar surface of foot	—	✓	✓

successful ways to massage this important lower body part. Please note that these photos are for demonstration purposes only, and the shorts worn by our model are longer than those you might ask a client to wear in order to receive deep tissue massage to the hip and thigh area. When treating the buttocks, adductors, hamstrings and quadriceps, it is helpful if the client wears running shorts (the kind with small slits at the sides). Be sure to use towels to drape your client in such a way that you expose as much as possible of the muscle you wish to work on while keeping the rest of the body covered.

Working with your client in the three-quarter-lying position affords you considerable leverage. In this position you may choose to treat either the limb positioned against the couch, or the limb resting uppermost. In the first six techniques discussed here we will treat the adductors, calf and Achilles tendon of a limb when it is against the couch. In the remaining techniques we will treat the lateral thigh—comprising the iliotibial band and vastus lateralis—plus the gluteals of the limb that is uppermost.

Using Your Forearms on Adductors

Step 1: To treat the right adductor muscles, position your client to be lying on her right side, with adductors clearly exposed.

Step 2: Taking care not to press into the popliteal space at the back of the knee, gently rest your forearm on the client and slowly but firmly glide towards the ischium.

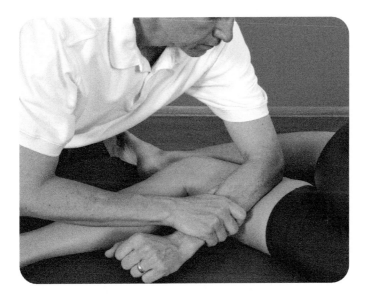

Advantages   The client is in a secure position and might feel less exposed than when adductors are treated in supine (compare this technique to the one on p. 131). ■ In this position the therapist has considerable leverage and can apply firm pressure to the adductor muscles of clients who require deep tissue massage in this area.

Disadvantage   For therapists to safeguard their own posture, they must stoop low to the treatment couch to perform this technique.

Using Your Elbows on Adductors

Step 1: To treat the right adductor muscles, position your client to be lying on her right side, with adductors clearly exposed.

Step 2: Taking care not to press into the popliteal space at the back of the knee, use a flexed elbow and, once again, slowly but firmly glide towards the ischium.

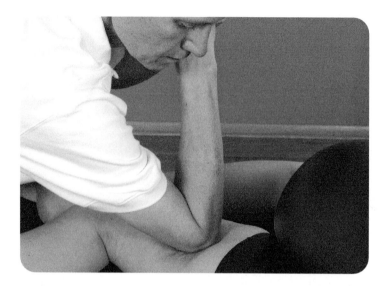

Advantages   Treating the adductors in this way facilitates access to the hamstrings. ▪ The client is in a secure position and might feel less exposed than when adductors are treated in the supine position.

Disadvantage   For therapists to safeguard their own posture, they must stoop low to the treatment couch to perform this technique.

Using Your Fists on Adductors

Step 1: To treat the right adductor muscles, position the client to be lying on her right side, with adductors clearly exposed. Ensure that the treatment couch is low enough for you to work with straight arms.

Step 2: Using your reinforced fist and keeping your wrists and elbows straight, press gently into the tissues; glide firmly from just above the popliteal space, working towards the ischium.

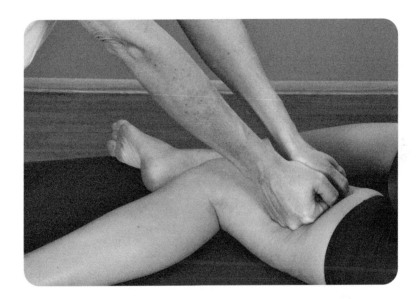

Advantage   This is a nice alternative to forearms and elbows; it allows you to treat from a more upright position yet still provide deep tissue massage.

Disadvantage   Therapists must avoid hunching their shoulders in an attempt to keep their arms straight and to avoid flexing their elbows.

Fisting the Medial Calf

Step 1: To treat the right calf muscles, position the client to be lying on her right side. Locate the Achilles tendon.

Step 2: With a reinforced fist, start where the calf muscles insert into the Achilles and glide firmly from this point to the medial side of the knee, compressing the tissues as you go.

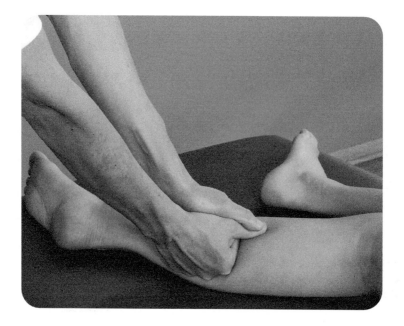

Advantage   This technique is great for accessing the medial side of the calf, a group of muscles usually only treated in prone or supine with the knee flexed.

Using Your Elbow on the Medial Calf

Step 1: To treat the right calf muscles, position your client to be lying on her right side. Locate the Achilles tendon.

Step 2: Touch the calf with your elbow and rest it there to apply localized pressure. Alternatively, use your elbow to glide slowly but firmly up the medial side of the calf in a continuous line. Remember to support yourself, perhaps by resting on the treatment couch, as shown.

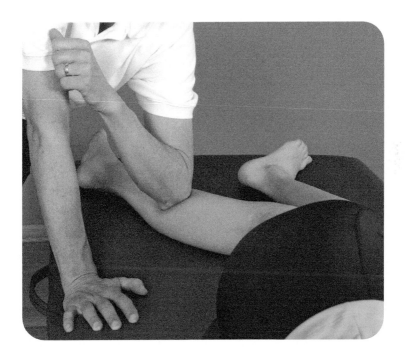

Advantages   This is a really deep technique useful for stubbornly tight calves. ▪ The technique is useful for deep pressure to specific areas of tightness.

Disadvantage   Because this technique is so powerful, be cautious not to go too deep too soon.

Treating the Achilles

Step 1: The Achilles is usually treated with the client prone, so it is useful to have an alternative position in which to apply your techniques. As for the treatment of the adductors and calf, position clients to be lying on their right side if this is the side you intend to treat.

Step 2: Sitting on the end of the treatment couch, flex the client's knee so you can support the ankle against your thigh. Work into and around the tendon, using your thumbs or by gripping the tendon and attempting to mobilize it.

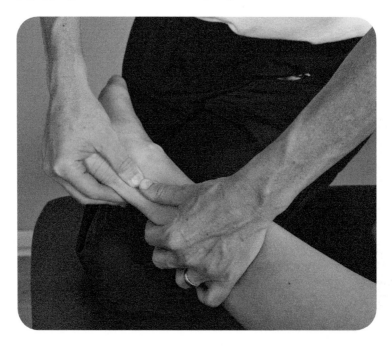

Advantage   This technique is a useful alternative to the prone position; it allows the therapist to access this large tendon in a different way, perhaps including massage to the medial side of the foot.

Disadvantage   Not all clients find this position comfortable.

CLIENT TALK

A female client who was keen on walking came to me for lower limb massage. She enjoyed receiving massage to her adductors and calves in three-quarter lying. I also included deep work around her Achilles tendon and foot in this position, because she had sprained her ankle many years previously and reported that the treatment provided relief to chronic achiness in the area.

Using Your Forearm on the ITB

Step 1: To treat a client's left lateral thigh in three-quarter lying, position the client so that this limb is uppermost.

Step 2: There are two ways you can use your forearm to apply deep tissue massage to this area. Standing so you are facing the front of the client, position your forearm just above the knee and, using your other hand for reinforcement, glide slowly and deeply up the lateral thigh, compressing the iliotibial band and vastus lateralis muscle.

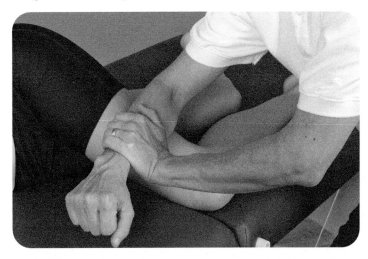

An alternative method is to stand behind the client and pull your forearm across the tissues, again from the knee to the thigh. Practice with both methods to see which you and the client find most effective.

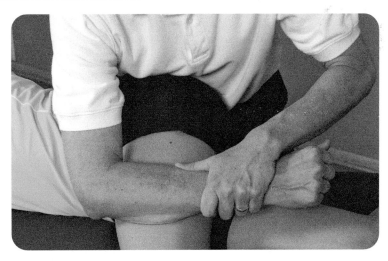

TIP Some clients feel more comfortable with a small folded towel or cushion beneath their knee on the side you are treating.

Advantage Both methods provide a good alternative to using palms for the treatment of vastus lateralis and this thick band of fascia.

Fisting the ITB

Step 1: Instead of using your forearms on the ITB, a stronger technique is to use reinforced fists. Begin with the client in three-quarter lying, and place your fists gently near the knee, avoiding bony structures.

Step 2: Keeping your wrists and elbows as straight as possible, glide firmly towards the hip.

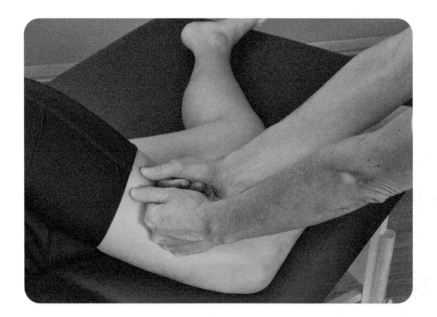

Advantage   This is a useful technique for working the distal end of the iliotibial band and vastus lateralis.

Disadvantage   It is difficult to maintain straight wrists and elbows all the way to the hip, so this technique might need to be reserved for small, distal points.

Applying Soft Tissue Release to the ITB

Step 1: You can enlist the assistance of your client with this technique. Position her in three-quarter lying, but this time with her uppermost knee slightly off the treatment couch.

Step 2: As you apply pressure with a reinforced fist, ask your client to slowly bend and straighten her knee as you glide 3 or 4 inches (7.5-10 cm) away from the knee, towards the hip. This produces an active-assisted stretch to the vastus lateralis muscle and, possibly, the iliotibial band.

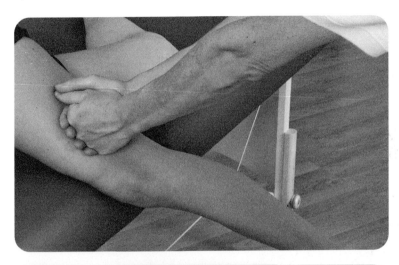

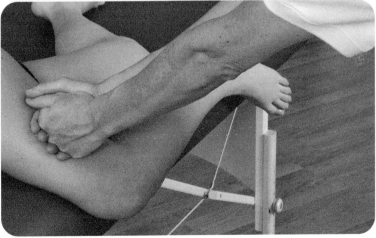

Advantage   This technique is reportedly very useful for clients with runner's knee and a very tight iliotibial band.

Disadvantage   This is not a particularly comfortable position for the client to remain in for very long.

Using Your Forearm on Gluteals

Step 1: A great way to alleviate tension in the gluteal area is simply to compress the tissues, focusing on areas of tightness. Working through a towel, start by working over the area consistently with your forearm, avoiding the use of elbows. (Here, the client is more side-lying than three-quarter lying. Three-quarter lying will give you better access to the gluteals. We also have removed the towel in this photo so you can see the area being treated more clearly.)

Step 2: You can continue to treat the area in this way, or you can apply a little oil, replace the towel and work over the area again. The oil will 'grip' the towel, and you can then use a twisting movement stretch as well as compress the tissues.

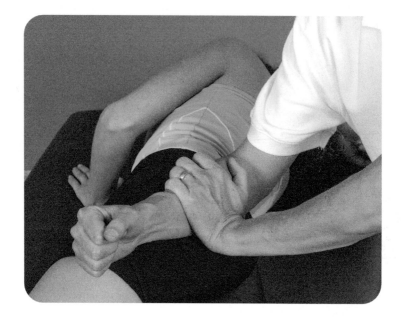

TIP A mistake some therapists make when treating gluteals is to use too much pressure too soon in too precise an area. In this position the client will sense the pressure far more than when prone.

Advantage This is a nice alternative to treating gluteals in prone and can be combined with treatment to the lateral thigh of the same limb, plus the tensor fascia latae muscle on this side as well.

Using Elbows on Gluteals

Step 1: Positioned as for the previous technique, using elbows is a way to focus pressure to more defined areas. Start by leaning onto the client, using your forearm to gauge their sensitivity to pressure.

Step 2: Should the client require deeper pressure, slowly flex your elbow. Remember that you need to flex your elbow only a few degrees for the client to experience a disproportionate rise in pressure.

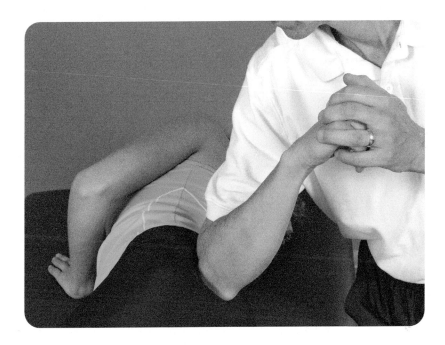

TIP Beware of deep pressure to the piriformis in this position because this can be painful—and discomfort does not necessarily indicate piriformis syndrome, as is believed by some therapists.

Advantages As an alternative to treating gluteals in prone, this technique can be combined with treatment to the lateral thigh of the same limb, plus the tensor fascia latae muscle on this side as well. ■ This technique is a great way to focus your pressure to localized areas.

Disadvantage This area is highly sensitive to pressure in many clients, so apply this technique cautiously.

Using Your Elbow on Tensor Fascia Latae

Step 1: This small muscle is much neglected by therapists yet seems to contribute to anterior and lateral thigh pain and to lateral knee pain. Your first step is to locate the muscle. In runners the muscle can be visibly identified, but this is not so in other clients. Like all muscles, it varies in size and slightly in shape.

Step 2: Apply static pressure to the muscle using your elbow.

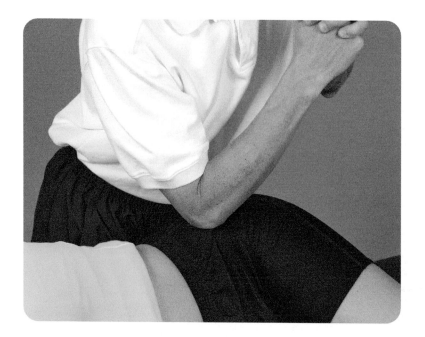

TIP To identify this muscle on clients, position them in supine and palpate the iliac crest. The muscle originates from the posterior aspect of the crest and will contract if you get clients to lift the leg off the treatment couch and rotate the hip internally. (You can try this yourself while standing: Flex your hip, keeping you knee straight, and internally rotate your hip.)

Advantage   This is a safe way to apply firm pressure to this small muscle.

Disadvantage   It can be difficult to identify the muscle if you are not accustomed to treating it in this position.

If you are a practicing therapist you likely are familiar with massaging the quadriceps and anterior leg with your client in supine position. You might even have learned to treat the adductors this way. Here we present techniques to treat the hamstrings and calf that prove useful when treating clients uncomfortable in the prone position.

Using Your Forearm on Hamstrings

Step 1: Try this unusual but effective way to treat hamstrings in supine. Start by positioning your client comfortably, in running shorts or in a towel draped to expose the area you intend to treat. Ask her to hold her leg as shown in the photo.

Step 2: Working from beneath the knee, lean into the tissues with your forearm, gliding towards the ischium.

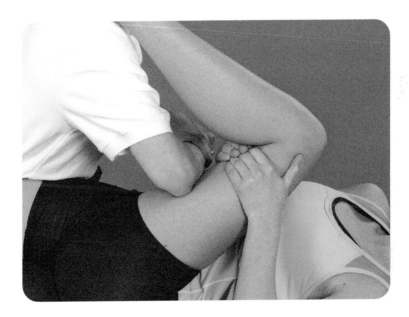

TIP If your client actively straightens the leg (maintaining hip flexion) as you glide from knee to ischium this acts like a form of active-assisted soft tissue release and is preferred by some clients.

Advantage   This technique is ideal for clients who cannot lay prone because of injury.

Disadvantages   It can be difficult to access the distal end of the hamstrings (near the knee) when the client holds her own limb. ■ This technique is not appropriate for all clients, some of whom might not want to hold their leg in this position.

Fisting Hamstrings

Step 1: Ensure the client is correctly draped in a towel, if necessary. Instead of the client holding her leg, practice resting the leg on your shoulder.

Step 2: Press your fist into the hamstrings, gliding from just below the knee to the ischium. Try to keep your wrist in a neutral position throughout.

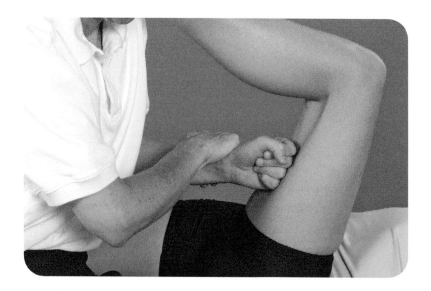

TIP If you choose to reinforce your fist, it is harder to get deep pressure than if you cup the knee with one hand while applying pressure with your other fist to prevent the client's hip from flexing further during the stroke.

Advantage   This technique is ideal for clients who cannot lay prone because of injury.

Disadvantages   It can be difficult to maintain your wrist in a neutral position while applying deep pressure. ■ This technique is not appropriate for all clients, some of whom might not wish to place their leg in this position.

Elbow Hamstrings

Step 1: Ask your client to hold her leg as shown; gently rest your elbow on her hamstrings.

Step 2: Working slowly, apply pressure to one spot, or slowly glide towards the ischium.

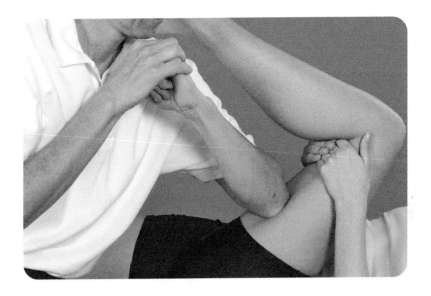

TIP To stretch the tissues as you compress them, ask your client to slowly straighten her leg, keeping her hip in this flexed position. This serves as an active-assisted stretch.

Advantages This technique is an excellent way to target tension in hamstrings, especially when combined with an active-assisted stretch. ■ This technique is ideal for clients who cannot lay prone because of injury.

Disadvantages This technique can be difficult to access the distal end of the hamstrings (near the knee) when the client holds her own limb. ■ The technique is not appropriate for all clients, some of whom might not wish to hold their leg in this position.

Calf Squeeze

Step 1: Flex your client's knee and gently sit on her foot to support the limb (otherwise she might try to keep the knee flexed rather than relaxing).

Step 2: Using oil, cup the distal end of the calf and squeeze it gently, allowing your palms to slide off the muscle, pulling it gently away from the bone. To assist venous and lymphatic drainage, work from the ankle to the belly of the muscle, to just below the knee, rather than from the knee to the ankle.

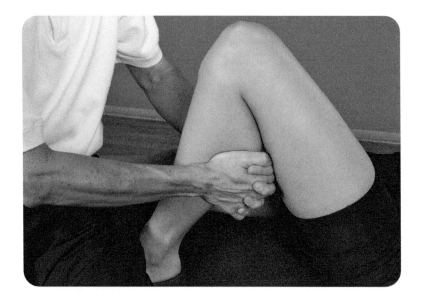

TIP This is a much more powerful technique than it might initially appear to be, so start gently and gradually build up the strength of your grip.

Advantages This technique is a nice way to treat the calf muscle in clients who cannot lay prone. ■ With the knee flexed and the ankle plantar flexed, the muscles of the posterior calf are in a passively shortened position; the gentle traction of these muscles away from the tibia feels pleasurable for most clients.

Using Your Forearm on the Calf

Step 1: Flex your client's knee and gently sit on her foot to support the limb (otherwise she might keep the knee flexed rather than relaxing). Use your forearms to effleurage from the ankle to below the knee. Practice pulling your forearm up and *across* the calf, sliding it from your elbow to wrist as you do so. Support the client's knee with your other hand.

Step 2: Change forearms and repeat the procedure.

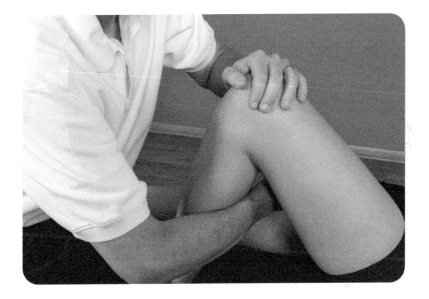

Advantages   This is a nice way to treat the calf muscle in clients who cannot lay prone. ▪ With the knee flexed and the ankle plantar flexed, the muscles of the posterior calf are in a passively shortened position; massage in this position feels pleasurable for most clients.

Using Your Forearm on the Quadriceps

Step 1: With the knee supported by a bolster, if necessary, apply oil either to the client or to your forearm; begin by resting gently just superior to the knee.

Step 2: Using a wide stance to protect your own posture, lean onto the client with your forearm as you slowly glide up the quadriceps. Start in the middle of the thigh, changing arms to massage the lateral thigh. (Note that your client will either need to wear shorter shorts or you'll need to towel drape in order to fully access the quadriceps.)

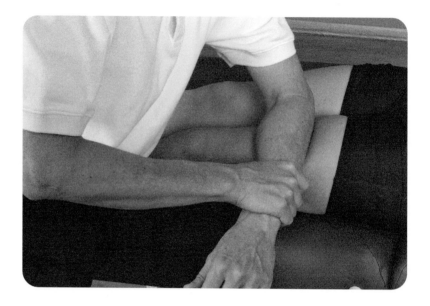

Advantage   This is a good deep tissue technique to follow petrissage to this area.

Quad Squeeze

Step 1: Kneeling down, if necessary, grip the quadriceps just above the knee and squeeze them away from the femur. Let your palms glide off the muscle as you do so.

Step 2: Continue to work this area of the quadriceps, moving towards the hip if possible.

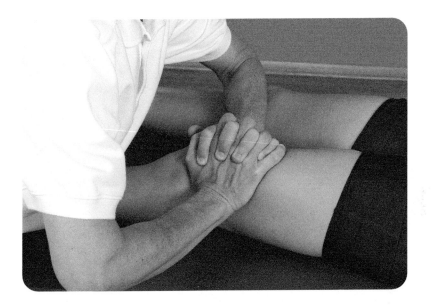

Advantage   This is an additional technique to have in your deep tissue toolbox.

Disadvantage   It can be difficult to work more than a limited area because your inside arm tends to encroach on the client's thigh that is not being worked as you move towards the hip.

Using Your Elbow on the Quadriceps

Step 1: With the client's knee supported with a bolster, if necessary, position your hand and elbow as shown in the photo.

Step 2: Using oil, apply pressure with your elbow, and use your hand to guide your elbow slowly up towards the hip. Take care that your guide hand does not encroach on the client's inner thigh.

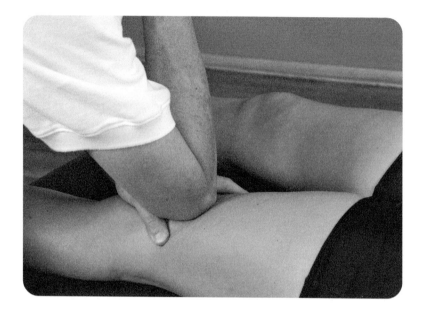

TIP The quadriceps can be bulky muscles, as you know, so don't be tempted to apply this technique without a guide hand because it can be difficult to stay in place.

Advantage   This is a great technique for applying deep and specific pressure to rectus femoris.

Disadvantage   It can be tricky to access the superior part of the rectus femoris without flexing the fingers of the guide hand to prevent intrusion in the groin area.

Fisting the ITB

Step 1: Lock your flexed elbow into your waist and position your fist just above the knee.

Step 2: Using oil, glide firmly towards the hip, compressing the lateral thigh. Reinforce your fist with your other hand—providing you have a wide stance and are not standing in unsupported flexion at the waist to perform the technique.

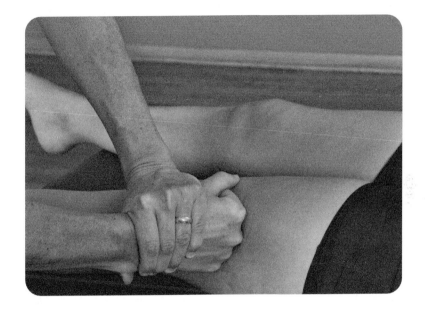

Advantage   This technique provides deep pressure to the lateral thigh.

Disadvantage   The technique can be tricky to perform if the treatment couch is not at the right height.

Using Your Forearm on the ITB

Step 1: Flex your client's knee and either sit on their foot or keep the limb in place using a soft bolster between the legs. Adduct your client's thigh.

Step 2: With oil, glide your forearm from just above the knee toward the hip, working over the lateral and anterolateral thigh.

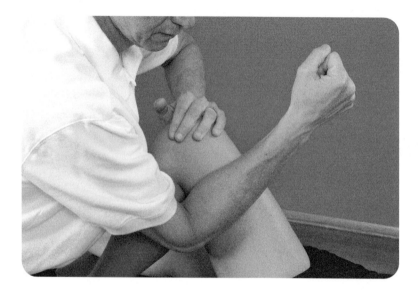

Advantage   This technique is an alternative way to apply firm pressure to the lateral thigh in supine.

Using Your Forearm on the Adductors

Step 1: With a low treatment couch, position your client so that her thigh is gently abducted and supported on your thigh, as shown (photo *a*). Use a folded towel under the client's leg (*b*) for support, if necessary. To treat the left adductors, use your left arm.

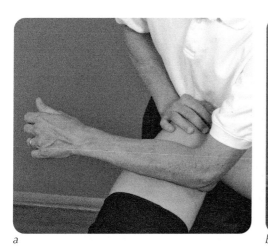 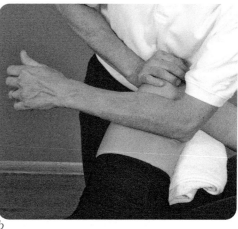

a　　　　　　　　　　　　　　　　*b*

Step 2: Starting just above the knee, glide your forearm slowly across the adductors towards the groin. Practice with your right arm (*c*) to see which you prefer using. (When using your right arm, notice where your hand ends up as you near the hip.)

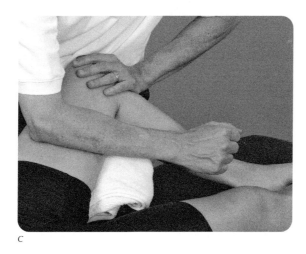

c

Advantage　This is a good way to access the adductors and perhaps do some specific work to the gracilis muscle.

Disadvantages　Some clients might feel a little too exposed in this position. ■ Not all therapists feel comfortable using their thigh as a support.

Applying Your Elbow to Tibialis Anterior

Step 1: Kneel at the end of the treatment couch. Position your client with her foot resting off the end of the treatment couch. Locate the tibialis anterior by asking your client to dorsiflex her foot and ankle. After locating the muscle, roll her leg inward so you have better access to the muscle.

Step 2: Using your elbow, press gently into the muscle just above the ankle and glide slowly towards the origin. The shin is a sensitive area for most clients, so little pressure is needed when using the elbow.

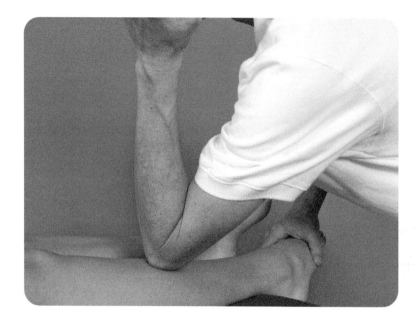

TIP By placing the foot over the end of the treatment couch, it is possible to passively turn the foot gently into inversion while applying this technique; this serves to stretch the fascia of the lateral and anterolateral leg. (Gently plantar flexing the client's ankle helps stretch the tibialis anterior.)

Advantage This technique is an easy way for the therapist to apply deep tissue massage to this muscle.

Disadvantage Not all therapists want to kneel down to perform this technique.

Knuckling Tibialis Anterior

Step 1: Stand at the end of the treatment couch. Position your client with her foot resting off the end of the treatment couch. Locate the tibialis anterior by asking your client to dorsiflex her foot and ankle. After locating the muscle, roll her leg inward so you have better access to the muscle.

Step 2: Use your knuckle to glide slowly up this muscle from just above the ankle to the origin of the muscle. Practice using one or more knuckles to find a comfortable method that works for you.

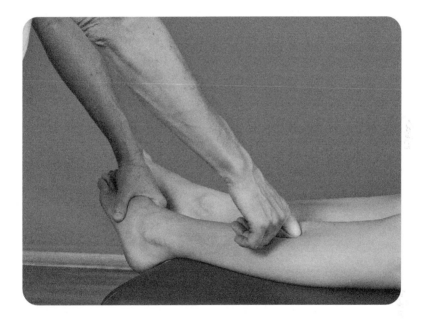

Advantage   The therapist does not need to kneel to perform this technique, which provides a much-needed alternative to therapists using their thumbs.

Disadvantage   Knuckles and thumbs are at risk of overuse.

Using a Tool on the Foot

Step 1: Pressure can be applied to the plantar surface of the foot by using a massage tool. Support the dorsal surface of the client's foot and, without oil, position the massage tool as shown in the photo.

Step 2: Apply gentle pressure to spots reported to feel beneficial by the client. Quite often this is on the medial aspect of the sole, along the course of the flexor hallucis longus muscle.

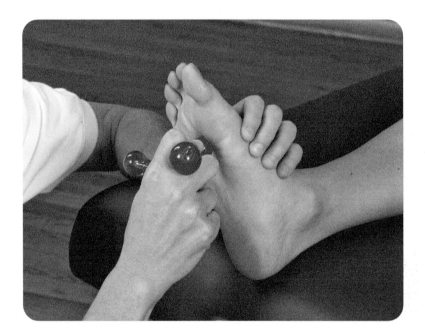

Advantage   This is a great technique to save therapists' thumbs and as an alternative to gentler techniques.

Disadvantage   Using a massage tool safely and effectively takes some practice; take care to press gently with this very localized form of pressure.

Treating Tensor Fascia Latae With a Tool

Step 1: Locate the tensor fascia latae by getting your client to raise her leg off the treatment couch, rotating it internally. Once located, position a massage tool gently against the muscle.

Step 2: Press firmly into the muscle, searching for trigger spots. When you locate one, apply gentle pressure for 60 seconds, allowing the 'grateful pain' to dissipate.

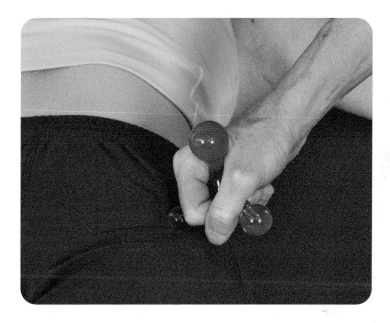

Advantage   This is a great technique to save therapists' thumbs when deep pressure needs to be applied to this small muscle.

Disadvantage   Using a massage tool safely and effectively takes some practice; take care to avoid pressure to the greater trochanter.

CLIENT TALK

A client who regularly ran half-marathons was treated with deep pressures to his tensor fascia latae muscle in supine. He arrived saying that the front of his hip just didn't feel right. As his case history was being taken, he explained how it felt better when he pressed 'here'. The spot he was pressing—and self-treating—was the tensor fascia latae muscle. After warming the area thoroughly, I applied deep pressures all over the muscle and gave him hip flexor stretches to do at home.

In this section you will practice deep tissue techniques with your client prone, a treatment position with which you are likely to be familiar. The main difference here is that for some techniques you will need to position clients with their feet off the end of the treatment couch.

Using Your Forearm on the Calf

Step 1: Position your client with her feet off the end of the treatment couch so she can dorsiflex at the ankle. Use your left arm to massage her right calf.

Step 2: Using oil, lean onto the client starting just above the Achilles, and glide slowly and firmly up the calf, stopping before you reach the popliteal space at the back of the knee. Notice that you can angle your forearm to redirect your pressure to the medial side of the calf using this arm, but to massage the lateral calf more firmly, you need to switch to your right arm, ensuring to keep your wrist and hand high so they do not intrude on the client's opposite leg.

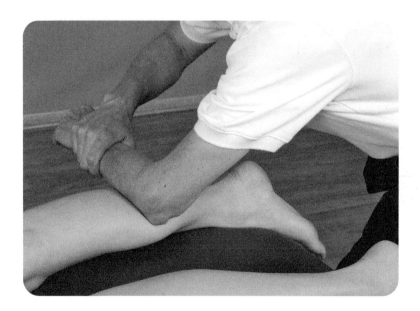

Advantages   This technique allows for really deep pressure to the calf. ■ The technique is easily linked to techniques that involve stretch as well as compression.

Disadvantages   Therapists need to remember to position clients with their feet off the couch when using this technique as part of an all-body treatment. ■ To protect their postures, therapists must stand in a wide stance or squat position.

Using Your Elbow on the Calf

Step 1: Position your client with her feet off the end of the treatment couch so she can dorsiflex at the ankle. Use your left arm to massage her right calf. Locate the Achilles tendon and place your elbow against the calf, supported by the web of your thumb.

Step 2: Start where the gastrocnemius and soleus muscles insert into the Achilles tendon. Using oil, glide firmly and slowly up the calf, using your hand to keep your elbow from slipping off the bulk of the muscle.

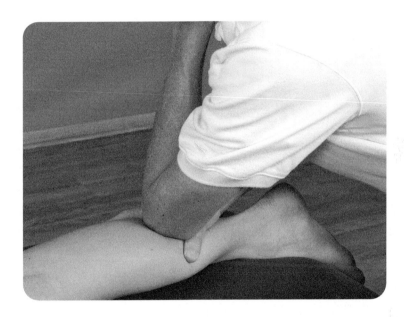

TIP To increase the intensity of the pressure, ask the client to dorsiflex her foot. This serves to lengthen the tissues on which you are working.

Advantages This is a really deep technique for clients who like deep pressure to this area. ■ This technique can be used to apply compression alone to a specific spot should this be required. ■ The technique is easily modified to increase the intensity of pressure.

Disadvantages Therapists need to remember to position clients with feet off the couch when using this technique as part of an all-body treatment. ■ To protect their postures, therapists must stand in a wide stance or squat position.

Fisting the Calf

Step 1: As an alternative to using your forearm or elbow, try this technique using reinforced fists. Position your client with feet off the end of the treatment couch and locate the Achilles tendon.

Step 2: Starting where the gastrocnemius and soleus muscles insert into the Achilles, press into the calf, gliding up the tissue and stopping before you reach the popliteal space at the back of the knee. Keep your elbows and wrists straight as far as possible. The therapist in the photo is using two hands. Practice what it feels like to press through a single fist, perhaps supporting your wrist with the other hand.

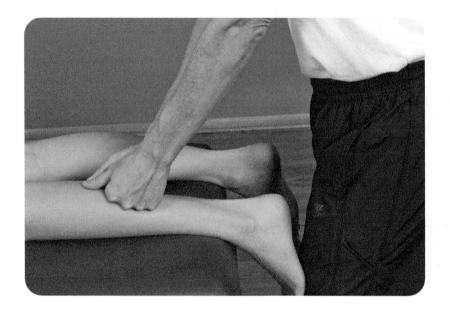

Advantage   This technique is easily modified to increase intensity of the pressure.

Disadvantages   Therapists need to remember to position clients with their feet off the couch when using this technique as part of an all-body treatment. ■ Unless the treatment couch is very low, it can be difficult for the therapist to maintain straight elbows and wrists.

Fisting the Calf With Dorsiflexion

Step 1: Try this enhanced fisting technique that helps to stretch tissues as they are being compressed. Passively dorsiflex your client's foot using your thigh, as shown in the photo. Locate the Achilles tendon.

Step 2: Starting where the gastrocnemius and soleus muscles insert into the Achilles, fist up the calf, *keeping the ankle in dorsiflexion*. Work the distal end of the calf in this manner rather than trying to massage all the way to the proximal end of the muscle. Because you are pressing through lengthened fibers, many clients experience a sensation of deep pressure even when pressure is fairly light.

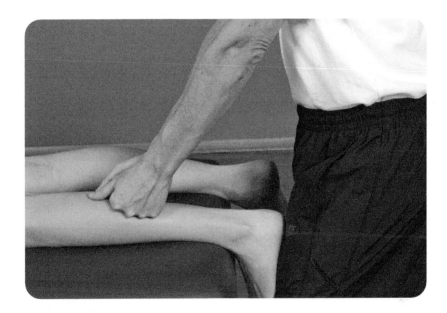

Advantage   This technique lets the therapist apply what for the client feels like very deep pressure.

Disadvantage   It can be tricky initially to learn to keep the ankle dorsiflexed while applying pressure with your hands.

Using Your Forearm to Apply Soft Tissue Release

Step 1: Now try a technique combining both pressure and stretch in a treatment that is a bit like the challenge of trying to pat your head at the same time as rubbing your belly. Flex the client's knee and support her ankle with your thigh, as shown. Practice dorsiflexing the client's ankle.

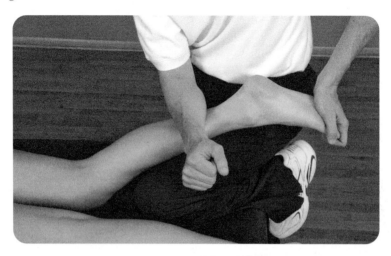

Step 2: Now comes the fun part! Using oil, practice your forearm technique while passively dorsiflexing the client's ankle. The trick with this technique is to dorsiflex the client's ankle three or four times *while maintaining the pressure of your forearm* and gliding from distal to proximal parts of the calf. Avoid pressure to the popliteal space at the back of the knee.

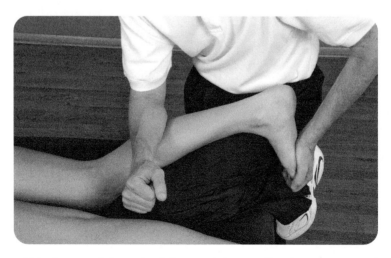

Advantage   This is a useful method for applying really deep pressure in an easily modifiable technique in a position that assists venous and lymphatic drainage of the leg.

Disadvantage   Not all therapists feel comfortable standing in this position to apply the technique.

Calf Squeeze

Step 1: Start by flexing your client's knee and resting it against your shoulder, passively shortening the calf muscles.

Step 2: Starting close to the Achilles tendon, squeeze the muscles away from the bone, working from the ankle towards the knee.

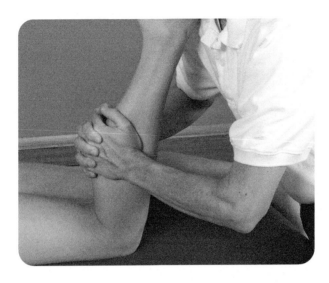

Advantages   The technique is easy to apply. ■ In this position the technique might aid venous and lymphatic drainage.

Disadvantage   The therapist must sit on the edge of the couch, albeit briefly, needing to twist at the waist.

Using Your Forearms on Hamstrings

Step 1: Ensuring to support yourself in flexion at the waist, position your forearm just above the knee. Use your left forearm to treat the client's right hamstring.

Step 2: Lean onto the client and glide firmly up to the ischium. End your stroke at that point on the thigh that is appropriate for your client. In sports massage, it is common to take the stroke all the way to the origin of the hamstrings at the ischium. In order to fully access these muscles, your client will either need to wear shorter shorts, or you'll need to provide towel draping.

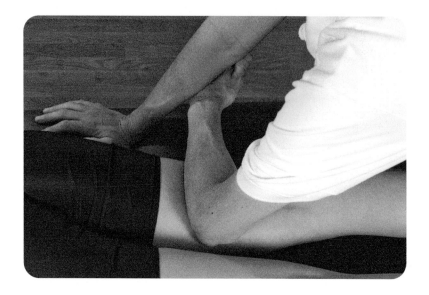

Advantage   This is an excellent way to apply deep tissue massage to the hamstrings in prone.

Disadvantage   Therapists must use a wide stance to prevent damage to their postures.

CLIENT TALK

I used deep tissue massage to the hamstrings in prone on a client who was a trapeze artist and, as part of his act, had to hang upside down with his knees hooked over the trapeze swing. He had consequently developed excessively tight muscles in both legs, which he found Swedish massage did little to alleviate. Initially, it was not possible to use elbows because the muscles were chronically tight, so forearms were used for many weeks, along with stretching techniques, before elbows could be introduced into the routine.

Using Your Elbows on Hamstrings

Step 1: Position your elbow just above the knee.

Step 2: Press into the tissues and glide slowly up the muscles towards the ischium. End your stroke at a point you feel is appropriate for your client, taking it all the way to the ischium if possible.

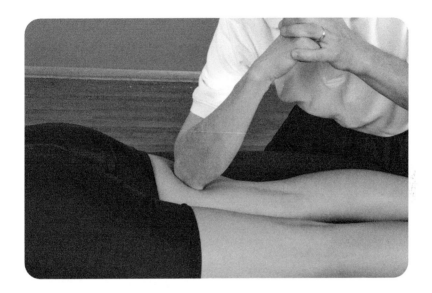

TIP If you have difficulty staying on the muscle in one continuous stroke, use the web of the thumb on your other hand as a guide for your elbow, but take care not to intrude on the inner thigh as the guide hand moves towards the hip.

Advantages   This technique is a method of applying really deep pressure to specific areas of the hamstring muscles. ▪ The elbow can be used to apply pressure to only specific areas of tension.

Disadvantage   Therapists must take a wide stance and take care to guard their own posture.

Working Into the Ischium

Step 1: Although not suitable for all clients, try this technique to apply deep pressure to the origin of the hamstrings. Position your client at the end of the treatment couch, resting on a pillow, if necessary. If needed, provide a stool on which your clients can rest their knees. Provide pillows to support their chest.

Step 2: Using your elbow, start a few inches (around 10 centimeters) distal to the ischium and glide slowly up the hamstrings until you feel the ischium beneath your elbow. This position cannot be maintained for more than two or three minutes, so only a few strokes are possible.

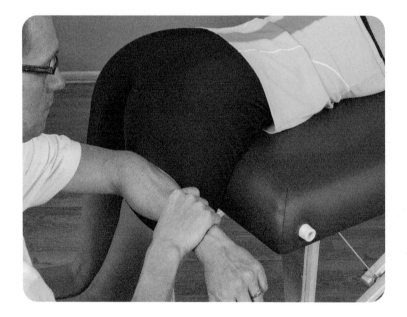

TIP If you can position clients in a kneeling position, this is more comfortable for them.

Advantage   This is an effective method of applying really deep pressure to the origin of the hamstrings.

Disadvantage   This technique may be used only with clients who feel totally comfortable in this unusual treatment position.

Accessing Piriformis

Step 1: To stretch the gluteal muscles, including the piriformis, place your elbow gently on the buttock, using a wide stance to protect your posture.

Step 2: While maintaining gentle pressure, move the hip between internal and external rotation. Note that as you move the client's foot towards you, you are rotating her femur internally; as you take her foot away from you, you are turning her femur externally.

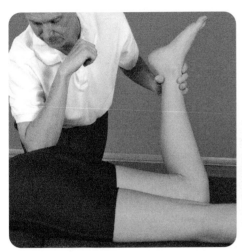 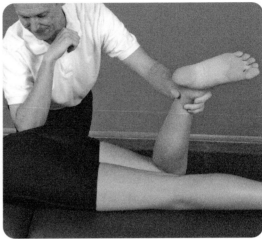

TIP The piriformis is sensitive in many clients because of its proximity to the sciatic nerve. Of course if you press onto the nerve, this will be uncomfortable. If your pressure is too deep, clients will simply contract their muscles, defeating your efforts. The trick with this technique is to work the area within the client's pain threshold *without* causing spasm in the muscles.

Advantages   This technique is effective for applying both compression and stretch to gluteals. ▪ It is easy to perform.

Disadvantage   Some clients find it difficult to 'let go' while having their hip moved in this way.

Fisting Tibialis Anterior

Step 1: Passively flex your client's knee.

Step 2: Starting at the ankle, use your fist to massage from the ankle to the knee. Little pressure is needed for this to feel 'deep'.

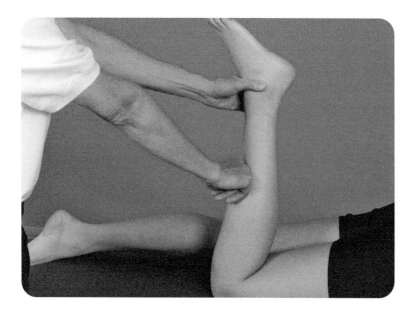

Advantage   This technique is useful for massaging the tibialis anterior, which is usually treated with the client supine.

Fisting the Foot

Step: Use your fist to compress the sole of the foot either with the foot flat on the couch, or as shown in the photo, while cupping the foot in your hand.

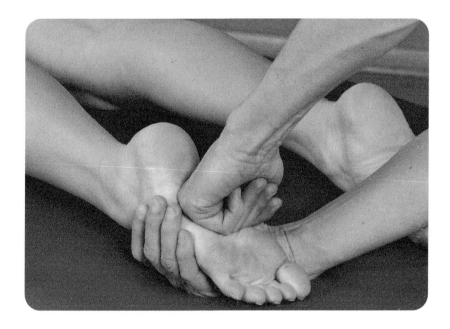

TIP If you find this technique is not strong enough, kneel down and practice compressing the tissues using your elbow.

Advantage This technique for treating the sole of the foot is especially useful on clients who are ticklish and for whom digital pressure is not tolerable.

Quick Questions

1. When treating the adductors in three-quarter-lying position, which other muscles are you able to access?

2. How can you introduce an element of stretch when treating hamstrings in supine using your forearm or elbow?

3. How do you locate the tensor fascia latae muscle to treat it in supine?

4. When squeezing the calf with the client prone, why do you work from the ankle to the knee?

5. If possible, to which bony structure should you end your stroke when treating hamstrings in prone with your elbow?

Deep Tissue Massage for the Upper Limbs

7

Using the three different treatment positions of three-quarter lying, supine and prone, the photographs and instructions in this chapter will teach you to apply deep tissue techniques to supraspinatus, infraspinatus, teres major and teres minor (see table 7.1). You will also learn how they can be used to treat the deltoid, biceps, triceps, wrist extensors and hand. As you know, latissimus dorsi acts powerfully on the shoulder joint, so it has been included here, where you will be introduced to some different techniques than those covered in chapter 5. We're going to start with a technique around the medial border of the scapula, which many therapists believe helps them access a very deep muscle, the subscapularis, by working through the rhomboid muscles.

Table 7.1   Muscles Targeted by Deep Tissue Massage Techniques Included in This Chapter

Muscle	POSITION		
	Three-quarter lying	Supine	Prone
Subscapularis	✓	—	—
Rhomboids	✓	—	—
Deltoid	✓	—	—
Latissimus dorsi	✓	—	—
Triceps	—	✓	✓
Teres muscles	—	✓	✓
Biceps	—	✓	—
Wrist extensors	—	✓	✓
Supraspinatus	—	—	✓
Infraspinatus	—	—	✓

Many techniques can be used in the three-quarter-lying position to apply deep tissue massage to the uppermost limb. In one of these techniques you can treat the limb against the treatment couch; we will begin with this one because it is unique.

Accessing Subscapularis

Step 1: For this treatment to work you need to modify the three-quarter-lying position so that your client is either lying on his arm or lies on his arm with his elbow flexed and behind him. On some clients the medial border of the scapula will become immediately apparent in either of these positions; in other clients, you might find it impossible to get really good access. If you can get your client into this position, the rhomboids will be passively shortened because the scapula has become passively retracted (adducted towards the spine).

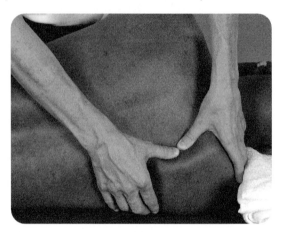

Step 2: When the medial border becomes apparent, as shown in the photo, simply press into it, using your thumbs. Ordinarily it is inadvisable for a therapist to press through an extended thumb joint, and you certainly should not do this if you are hypermobile. However, the leverage you have in this position is so great that very little pressure is required to push into the rhomboid muscles in this way. Compare this treatment to the supine technique described on page 156.

Usually, subscapular techniques are attempted with the client in the prone position. Many therapists believe that pressing through the middle fibers of the trapezius and rhomboids to get under the medial border of the scapula gives them access to the subscapularis. What do you think?

> ### CLIENT TALK
>
> I used this method indirectly when approached by two therapists who frequently exchanged treatments with each other. A male therapist, a bodybuilder with a large frame, complained that his girlfriend, of much smaller frame, could never quite 'get into' the tension he felt in his rhomboids. After experimenting with the deep tissue techniques to this area described in chapter 5, I showed his girlfriend this unusual treatment position, which both she and her boyfriend much preferred.

Advantage   This technique is an alternative method of applying pressure to the rhomboid muscles and to this region of the scapula; it can be useful when other methods have failed.

Disadvantages   Not all clients feel comfortable lying in this position. ■ The position cannot be maintained for long.

Using Your Forearm on Deltoids

Step 1: Chronic tension in the deltoid muscle can be tricky to treat. Try holding your client's uppermost arm to prevent movement; position your forearm at the insertion of deltoid.

Step 2: Glide firmly across the muscle, gliding off the head of the humerus. Use your elbow to apply pressure to specific areas of tension on the muscle.

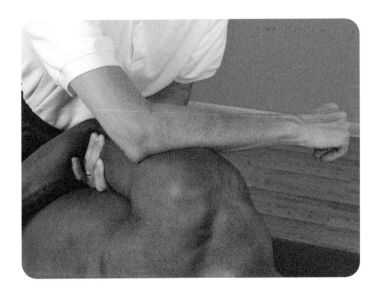

Advantage   This technique provides powerfully deep massage to this muscle.

Disadvantage   Clients can sometimes feel they are being squashed as the therapist leans on them in this position.

Applying Pressure to Latissimus Dorsi

Step 1: Have your client take his arm above his head, lengthening the latissimus dorsi muscle.

Step 2: Starting at the shoulder, reinforce your palms and lean onto the client as you glide firmly over this small area. In this position you have access not only to latissimus dorsi but to the origin of the triceps muscle, which can be tender, so work with caution.

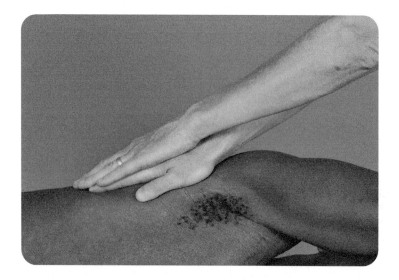

Advantage   This is a great technique for applying deep tissue massage to clients with tight adductor muscles or who frequently use their triceps as part of their sport or hobby.

Treating the Posterior Shoulder

Step 1: For more specific pressure to this area, practice using your elbow, locating the spot gently to begin, supporting the client's arm, as shown in the photo.

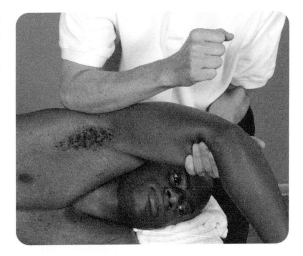

Step 2: Slowly flex your elbow, localizing the pressure. Note that little force is needed because this area is rarely included in massage treatment and might be sensitive.

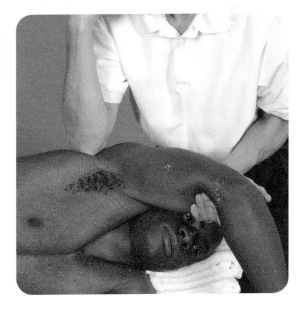

Advantages   This technique is easily incorporated with techniques for the trunk performed in three-quarter lying. ■ The technique is a useful addition to a therapist's set of skills for treating the shoulder, as this area is much neglected.

Disadvantage   The technique can be tiring to perform on clients with very heavy arms.

Try these deep tissue techniques that can be easily incorporated into your existing massage routine.

Using Your Forearm on Triceps

Step 1: Take your client's arm above his head, using your thigh for support.

Step 2: Starting at the elbow, lean onto the client and glide your stroke towards—and even over—the armpit, but avoid localized pressure to the armpit itself. The best way to apply this technique is to use your left arm when treating the client's right triceps. Notice where your hand ends up if you attempt the technique using your right hand.

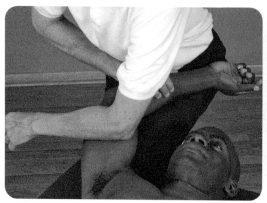 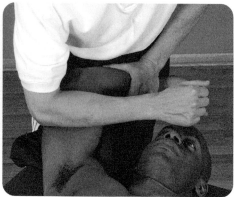

TIP You will find this technique much easier if you work with a low treatment couch.

Advantages   This technique is easily incorporated into a massage routine. ▪ It is a good way to apply deep tissue massage to the triceps muscle.

Disadvantage   Some therapists feel uncomfortable using their thigh to support the client's limb.

CLIENT TALK

A tennis player enjoyed receiving treatment to his triceps muscles in this position. He had large, bulky triceps, and I found it much easier to apply deep tissue massage to these muscles using my forearm in this supine position than I did performing petrissage to the muscles in prone. Gripping the muscles using petrissage was difficult because of their size and increased tone, so it was a relief to be able to apply the firm, broad compression afforded by this technique.

Fisting Triceps

Step 1: Hold your client's arm, supporting the arm at the elbow, as shown.

Step 2: Using your fist, press into the triceps muscle, working from the elbow to the armpit. Avoid deep localized pressure into the armpit in this position.

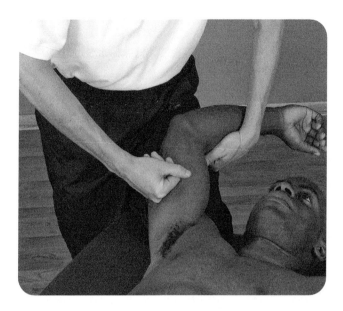

TIP If you apply gentle traction to the arm as you glide, you are adding a stretch component to your treatment.

Advantages This technique is easy to incorporate with a regular massage routine. ▪ You can vary the position of your fist to access the fibers of pectoralis major.

Disadvantage It can be tiring to treat clients with heavy arms using this technique.

Accessing the Lateral Border of the Scapula

Step 1: Holding your client's arm in this abducted position, locate the lateral border of the scapula at the point where the teres major and teres minor muscles originate.

Step 2: Using your knuckle, press onto these muscles and even onto the anterior surface of the scapula in an attempt to access subscapularis. Avoid localized pressure into the armpit itself. Little pressure is needed to press along this bony border.

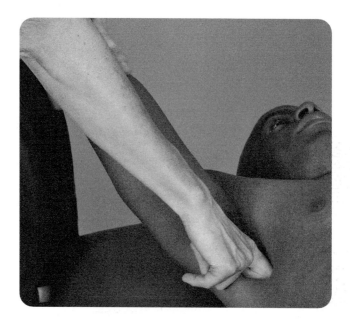

Advantages This technique is useful in applying deep pressure to the teres major and teres minor muscles, which are often neglected in a massage sequence. ■ Some therapists believe this technique helps them access the subscapularis muscle.

Disadvantage Using knuckles is not ideal because it is difficult to keep the finger joints in alignment.

Fisting Biceps

Step 1: For clients who require deep pressure to their biceps, try fisting the tissue in addition to your petrissage techniques. Holding the client's wrist, start your stroke just above the elbow.

Step 2: Lean onto the muscle through your fist as you glide slowly up the muscle towards the shoulder. Notice that if you apply gentle traction to the arm, you are adding a stretch component to this compressive technique. However, to do this, try to hold the client on or superior to the wrist joint so you are mostly tractioning the elbow.

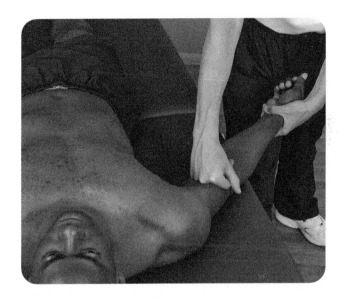

Advantages   This is an additional technique for treating clients who like deep pressure but who perhaps have large and bulky biceps muscles that are difficult to petrissage. ■ Traction can easily be added to stretch the tissues.

Disadvantage   Therapists need to take care to traction the elbow only and not the wrist as well.

Fist Wrist Extensors

Step 1: Support your client's forearm on a towel if necessary.

Step 2: Starting just superior to the wrist joint, fist slowly and deeply up the extensor muscles to the elbow, avoiding the lateral epicondyle of the humerus. Notice that you can greatly increase your pressure if you change the part of your fist you are using. In the photo, the therapist is using his phalangeal bones pressed flat against the skin; if you make a firm fist, you can get deeper pressure by running your proximal interphalangeal joints across the tissue.

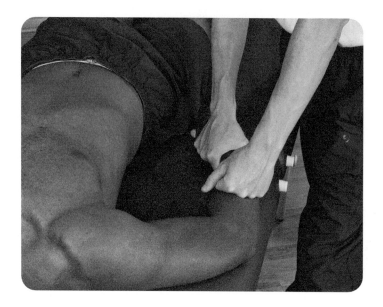

TIP As an alternative, you can kneel down (or take a really wide stance) facing your client and practice running *your* right forearm across the client's right forearm extensors.

Advantage This technique is easy to apply and incorporate into a regular massage routine.

Fisting the Palm

Step 1: It is tempting to use our fingers and thumbs to treat the hands of our clients. We will always need to apply massage in this way to some areas of the body, but the more techniques we can adopt to avoid this practice the better. Working on the hand is a good place to start. Cup the client's hand in a way that is comfortable for you both. In the example shown, the therapist has chosen to sit on the edge of the treatment couch and is resting the client's hand on a folded towel.

Step 2: Supporting the client's palm in your hand, as shown, gently fist into it, stretching and compressing the tissues as you twist the skin. Notice that you need almost no oil on this area. Fist into the thenar and hypothenar eminences of the palm, abducting the client's thumb to help stretch the thenar eminence. Alternatively, ask the client to really extend his fingers as you fist into the palm. Work the fleshy areas only, avoiding direct pressure to the knuckles and finger joints.

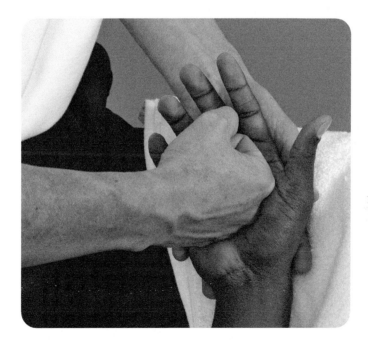

Advantage   This technique is a good way to practice working on a small area without using your fingers and thumbs.

Squeezing the Palm

Step: Practice squeezing your client's hand between your own, working your palms into the fleshy parts of his hand.

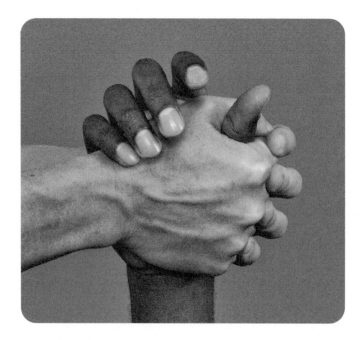

Advantage   This is an added technique to help you avoid the temptation of always using your fingers and thumbs to treat small areas.

Here are some additional deep tissue techniques you might not have come across for treating the upper limb in prone.

Accessing Supraspinatus

Step 1: This technique is great for applying localized deep pressure to fleshy muscles of the neck and shoulder. When treating the supraspinatus, for example, you will also be treating the upper fibers of the trapezius, through which you need to press. Locate the supraspinatus and gently place a massage tool at the spot at which you want to apply pressure. A massage tool may be used equally well on the trapezius.

Step 2: Apply pressure to those areas that provide most relief from tension for your client. Clients should report feeling that 'grateful pain' sensation that is tolerable and which eases within a few minutes. Remove the massage tool and soothe the area with effleurage or petrissage before repeating in the same place or moving to another spot.

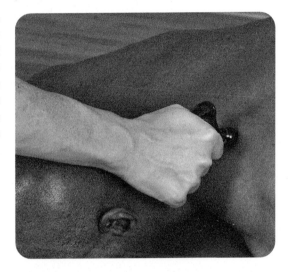

TIP To locate the supraspinatus in prone, find the bony V shape formed where the spine of the scapula meets the acromion process.

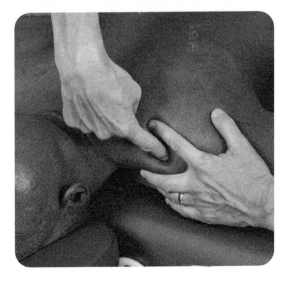

Advantage This technique is a brilliant way to get therapists out of the habit of using their thumbs to apply deep localized pressure to this area. ■ Most clients cannot tell the difference between pressure from a massage tool and the pressure of a therapist's thumb.

Disadvantage It takes a little practice to get used to using a massage tool.

Finding the Teres Muscles

Step 1: As a starter for working this sensitive area in prone, practice locating the lateral border of the scapula with the client's arm abducted as you kneel by the side of the treatment couch. Here you can access the teres major and teres minor muscles as well as the triceps and the posterior fibers of the deltoid muscle.

Step 2: Reinforce your thumbs to apply gentle pressure all around this area.

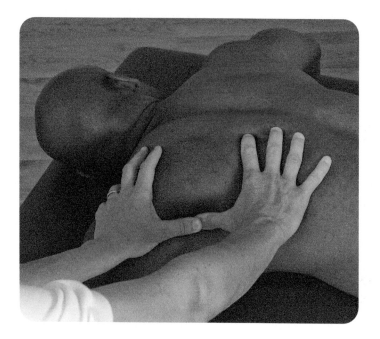

Advantage   This technique is easy to apply to this much-neglected area, with little pressure required.

Disadvantages   The technique needs to be used selectively because continued pressure through the thumb joint in this position is not advisable. ■ Not all therapists want to kneel to perform this technique.

Working the Posterior Shoulder

Step 1: Kneeling at the side of the treatment couch, gently abduct the client's arm.

Step 2: Using oil, glide across the proximal aspect of the triceps muscle and into the back of the shoulder. If this feels like it might be too severe, simply use your forearm to glide across the triceps, compressing the tissues in a form of deep effleurage.

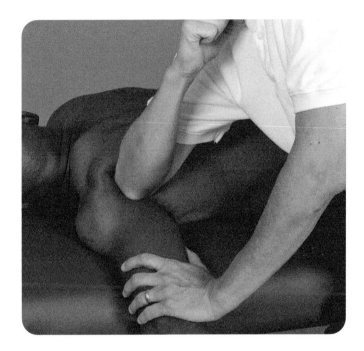

Advantages   This technique is easily incorporated into a massage routine. ■ It is easily modified to allow you to use your elbow or forearm. ■ Gentle traction can be used at the same time as the application to further stretch the tissues.

Disadvantage   Not all therapists feel comfortable kneeling to perform this technique.

Tractioning the Glenohumeral Joint

Step 1: This technique is great for both compressing and stretching the tissues around the glenohumeral joint. Start by kneeling at the side of the treatment couch, supporting the client's arm in abduction.

Step 2: Pressing though your palm, traction the joint at the same time. With practice, you can glide your palm up the triceps from the elbow, all the while applying gentle traction, ending your stroke on the back of the armpit.

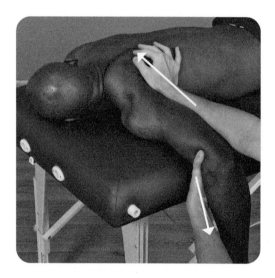

TIP For really deep pressure and stretch, apply a little oil and then place a facecloth over the area. Perform the technique through the facecloth, turning your hand to stretch and compress the tissues simultaneously.

Advantage   This technique is an easy way to stretch and compress the tissues of this part of the shoulder.

Disadvantage   Not all therapists feel comfortable kneeling to perform this technique.

Using Your Forearm on Wrist Extensors

Step 1: Kneeling at the top of the treatment couch, position the client as shown in the photo, with his wrist slightly over the edge of the couch.

Step 2: Use your forearm to gently compress the tissues as you glide from the wrist to the elbow. Notice how you can modify the intensity of the compression if you extend and flex the client's wrist over the edge of the couch while stroking with your forearm. This is similar to the technique used on page 140, where, in prone, the client has his ankle dorsiflexed at the same time as the therapist runs his forearm across the calf muscles.

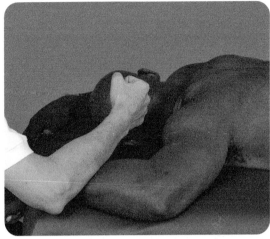

Advantage   This technique is an easy way to apply firm pressure to the extensor muscles of the forearm in prone.

Disadvantage   Not all therapists feel comfortable kneeling to perform this technique.

CLIENT TALK

With the client in prone, I used this method of treating the wrist extensor muscles when working with a client who was a keen motorcyclist. He traveled many miles on his bike and often suffered from tension in his forearms because of the posture necessary for riding. He much preferred to receive deep tissue massage to his forearms in prone, which he felt was more beneficial than when he received the treatment in supine.

Using Your Elbow on Infraspinatus

Step 1: Infraspinatus originates from the infraspinous fossa on the posterior scapula, as you know. It often contains sensitive trigger points, especially in the very centre of the muscle. Locate one of these points and gently position your elbow there.

Step 2: Slowly lean onto the point, noting that very little pressure is required. Remain there for around a minute—enough time for any client discomfort to dissipate. Soothe the area and repeat in the same or a different spot. Remember that if the client tenses, your pressure is too deep, so soothe the area and start again.

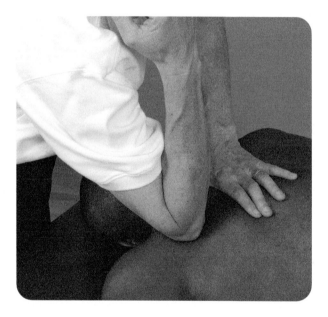

Advantage   This technique is a nice way to add deep tissue massage to a muscle that is usually treated only with effleurage in Swedish massage routines.

Disadvantage   It can take practice to locate the trigger spots in this muscle.

Quick Questions

1. Through which other muscles do you need to press in an attempt to access the subscapularis muscle in the three-quarter-lying position?

2. When treating triceps in supine using either your forearm or fist, to which structure should you avoid localized deep pressure?

3. What two techniques can you employ to treat the hand of a client in supine to help you avoid using your own fingers and thumbs on this area?

4. How do you locate the supraspinatus muscle with the client in prone position?

5. What should you do if your client tenses while you are applying pressure to the infraspinatus muscle in prone?

PART IV

Deep Tissue Massage Routines and Programmes

We have come to the practical application of the techniques you have learned as they relate to your massage practice. Selected compressive and stretching techniques from previous chapters are sequenced here to form practice routines. These routines are examples of how you might incorporate your new techniques into a full body massage in the three-quarter, supine or prone position. Also here is information on taking a case history from clients, including questions that relate particularly to the application of deep tissue massage. Overviews of three case studies illustrate the scope for the use of this form of massage. The routines presented here are designed to be illustrative rather than prescriptive; they demonstrate just some of the ways the techniques you have learned in chapters 5, 6 and 7 can be applied. Use the ideas in this part of the book to help you structure and develop your own routines, selecting from the book those techniques you enjoy and find most helpful.

8

Creating Deep Tissue Massage Routines

In this final chapter we begin with some questions you might wish to ask potential clients to ascertain whether deep tissue massage is appropriate for them. After that, we look at some pointers to help you get to grips with performing this type of massage within a regular treatment time. The bulk of the chapter provides suggested practice sequences for treating clients in three-quarter-lying, supine and prone positions. You can use these sequences as a starting point, and modify them when you feel ready, selecting techniques from earlier chapters. As examples of how deep tissue massage can be applied in real-life situations, we will look at three case studies: a female bodybuilder, a serious runner and a client recovering from a wrist injury.

Initial Questions

As you will discover from reading the case studies later in the chapter, not all clients approach a therapist seeking deep tissue massage. In many cases, it is the therapist rather than the client who decides that this form of massage might be more beneficial than general Swedish massage—that it might result in a better treatment outcome. When a client specifically requests deep tissue massage, there are some questions you should ask prior to treatment, in addition to those questions you normally ask when taking your client's medical history. You will not want to ask all these questions of all clients, and you should adapt them to each situation. Select from these questions the ones that are relevant to your client and feel free to phrase them in your own words.

TIP For more information on how to take a client medical history, see *Soft Tissue Release* (J. Johnson, 2009, Champaign, IL: Human Kinetics).

The first six questions pertain to new clients who have had deep tissue massage before; the seventh question should be asked of all clients wanting deep tissue massage.

1. Why did you have deep tissue massage?

   With this question you are trying to determine why the client wants deep tissue massage *again* and what their expectations might be of the deep tissue massage treatment you will provide. Do they want deep tissue massage because they previously found it pleasurable? Or simply because they always have this type of massage? Or do they think they ought to have deep tissue massage because the last therapist they saw told them it was a good treatment for a particular condition they have? This last reason is quite common in clients seeking treatment for the rehabilitation of sporting injuries. Often another therapist has indicated that the only real solution to very tight muscles or a tight iliotibial band is deep tissue massage.

2. Who performed the massage and for what reason?

   Knowing who performed the treatment and why is helpful. Was treatment for a particular condition, such as a restricted joint or particularly tight-feeling muscle? If so, is this what the client wants to have treated again? Or was deep tissue massage simply the preference of the previous therapist?

3. How was the massage applied?

   Although you cannot replicate the exact treatment style and routine of another therapist, and might not wish to, knowing when something worked well comes in handy. Was application part of an oil massage? Or was it through clothing as part of a seated chair massage routine?

4. Was this a recent treatment or did they receive it some time ago?

   When did the client receive the treatment? Last week? Last month? Last year? If the treatment was a long time ago, say, over a year, and the client has not received a treatment since, why? Was he or she too busy? Was there an illness or a contraindication? Or did something put the client off having massage again? When clients receive their first deep tissue treatment from a therapist who believes in the no-pain-no-gain approach, they might come away feeling this form of massage was too deep. They might have even suffered bruising. If so, they are understandably reluctant to repeat the experience, no matter how badly they feel they need treatment. It might take them months or longer before they seek treatment from another therapist. In such a case, you know you have to pay special attention to gaining and maintaining rapport with the client, reassuring him or her that deep tissue massage need not be painful. Conversely, you might meet a client who has enjoyed deep tissue massage. In either case, you will want to solicit more information about the treatment itself.

5. How did the previous treatment feel? Did they enjoy it?

   If a client has had deep tissue treatment before and enjoyed it, you can try to repeat that treatment or even improve on it. The more information you can discover about the treatment, the better. Was it deep enough? Did any aspect of the treatment feel too deep? Were there aspects they particularly liked or disliked? If a client answers, 'I loved it, but it was painful on my legs', this prompts further questions. What does the client mean by 'legs'—the regions from the knees to the ankles, as defined in anatomy, or the whole of the lower limb? Was it the front or the back of the legs or both that were painful? Clients often provide a lot of information in one answer. For example, they might say, 'It hurt on the front of my leg, here, and the therapist said that it might be because I'd been running a lot this week, and when I told him it hurt, he did it less hard. It was okay after that.' From this kind of information there is much to glean that can be helpful to you in the future.

6. How did the client feel following treatment?

We all hope our clients express positive feelings following treatment, saying things like, 'I felt great. Everything felt better, and my shoulders were no longer stiff.' You don't want to prompt the client but do also need to know if they experienced adverse effects such as bruising, DOMS or lightheadedness. If they report, 'It was ok, but I felt sore for a few days', this raises the question, 'Why are you returning for deep tissue massage?' Do they want to feel sore? Do they think they need to feel sore for the treatment to be effective? Or are they hoping to enjoy the sensation of deep tissue massage this time without feeling sore again afterwards?

7. What do you want from *this* treatment?

Does the client want deep tissue massage on all parts of the body? Or are there parts of the body to which they don't want to receive deep tissue massage? (See case study A, p. 193, for an example of a client who had preferences such as this.) Having read the safety guidelines on page 24, you will know there are some areas or structures to which deep tissue techniques should not be applied. However, the client might report disliking massage when applied to their quadriceps but liking it when applied to their hamstrings.

Tests

If you are using deep tissue massage as part of a programme to help improve the range of motion in a joint, you will find it helpful to first assess this range, then perform your treatment using deep tissue techniques (plus other modes of treatment, perhaps), and then to reassess the joint. Which tests you perform obviously depends on the joint you are treating. If it is the knee joint, for example, you will need to test flexion and extension; if it is the ankle, you will need to test plantar flexion and dorsiflexion as well as inversion and eversion.

Most textbooks on musculoskeletal assessment include information on joint testing. To discover normal joint ranges, refer to *The Clinical Measurement of Joint Motion*, edited by Walter B. Greene and James D. Heckman and published by the American Academy of Orthopaedic Surgeons.

Notes Concerning Timing

Most Swedish massage treatments last an hour. With slow, controlled holds, strokes and stretches, deep tissue massage takes longer to apply. If you were to employ all the techniques in chapters 5 (the trunk), 6 (the lower limbs) and 7 (the upper limbs), delivering them slowly and conscientiously as necessary, your treatment would last a very long time indeed. You might be tempted to rush the strokes, applying them with the same pace as Swedish massage, but this would be counterproductive and would likely cause pain. How do you handle the timing issue, then? You have at least three possibilities:

- Agree to treat the whole body in a single session but to provide deep tissue techniques to only one part of the body, such as the backs of the legs. This is a good idea particularly when you are first starting to incorporate the techniques with your treatment.

- Treat only one part of the body during a single treatment session. This is useful when the client wants only that part treated anyway, or when there is a particular problem to address (such as a stiff neck and shoulders). Take care, however, to avoid overworking that area.

- Provide a massage of a longer duration. This is not always possible for the client or the therapist and is of course more expensive for the client. Plus, a longer treatment might not be beneficial from a physiological point of view. Deep tissue massage for 90 to 120 minutes can leave a client feeling exhausted rather than relaxed. However, some therapists offer longer treatments that are attractive and appropriate for some clients.

As you learned in chapter 2 (p. 32 Top Tips for Treating Clients), whether a client 'switches off' immediately, or more gradually as the treatment progresses, there is a palpable decrease in the tone of their muscles at the end of a treatment compared to at the beginning. You do not need to use as much pressure towards the end of a treatment because by this time tissues are usually fairly pliable.

Two other interesting observations are, first, that clients appear to become acclimatized to deep tissue massage with subsequent treatments—their tolerance to pressure increases. Second, their bodies seem to respond more favourably. As you compress trigger points, for example, the decrease in tone occurs far more readily than when you first started using compression with this client.

TIP Providing your clients with active stretches they can do at home will dramatically improve treatment outcomes if these outcomes involve wanting to overcome muscle imbalance or improve posture. Deep tissue massage helps stretch and lengthen muscles, but its effects are countered when the client readopts the very posture that is causing the problem. Asking clients to change their posture and to do some stretches for those muscles is a helpful adjunct to your treatments.

Practice Routines

Massage is a flowing, organic therapy, as you know, and to try to pigeon hole therapists into performing a set routine would be unwise. You probably massage differently
from your colleagues, perhaps despite similar training, and work with what feels most
comfortable and natural to you. The routines presented here are designed to help you
practice the techniques as part of an integrated treatment rather than as disparate or
isolated steps. If you don't like a particular step, leave it out. As you work through each
routine, practice applying each technique, and also practice linking the techniques
together using the strokes you regularly use. Remember that full instructions (with tips)
for all these techniques can be found in chapters 5, 6 and 7.

Many therapists initially find deep tissue techniques awkward to apply smoothly and
consistently because many of the techniques involve moving the client's limbs, and
most therapists are accustomed to treating clients in prone or supine positions with
little movement involved. With practice, you will discover that it is easy to passively
move a client's limbs, and that the limbs remain perfectly relaxed as you do this. Part
of the reason for including these routines here is to help you practice how to pick up,
hold and move a limb in a way that feels comfortable for both you and your client.

You will want to know how long it takes to perform each of these steps within the
routines provided. Suggested times are given as rough guides only. You might find it helpful to complete the Routine Checklist on pages 176-177. After completing the checklist,
you can assess your findings and select the techniques you will start incorporating into
your own treatments, adapting them to the needs of your clients.

TIP   Keep oil and a facecloth (or small towel) within easy reach at all times. You might find it
helpful to have a small cushion on which to kneel while applying some of the techniques.
You will also want a massage tool with which to practice compression of certain muscles.

ROUTINE CHECKLIST

You might find it helpful to complete the checklist on pages 176-177 as you work through
each of the practice routines. When you have finished, identify those techniques you liked,
those that you wish to drop, those that took longer to apply than others and so on. Notice
that we have left space for your comments for both the left (L) and right (R) sides of the body
because you might find that applying a technique to one side of the body is different from
applying it to the other. In such a case, you need to ask yourself what you might be doing
differently the second time around.

Position	Time taken	Comments
Three-quarter lying		
1. Using Your Forearm on Upper Trapezius		L: R:
2. Using Your Elbow on Levator Scapulae		L: R:
3. Stretching Latissimus Dorsi		L: R:
4. Treating the Posterior Shoulder		L: R:
5. Using Your Forearm on Quadratus Lumborum		L: R:
6. Using Your Elbow on Quadratus Lumborum		L: R:
7. Treating the Achilles		L: R:
8. Fisting the Medial Calf		L: R:
9. Using Your Elbow on the Medial Calf		L: R:
10. Using Your Forearms on Adductors		L: R:
11. Using Your Forearm on the ITB		L: R:
12. Using Your Forearm on Gluteals		L: R:
Supine		
1. Applying Your Elbow to Tibialis Anterior		L: R:
2. Using Your Forearm on the Quadriceps		L: R:
3. Using Your Forearm on the ITB		L: R:
4. Using Your Forearm on the Adductors		L: R:
5. Calf Squeeze		L: R:
6. Using Your Forearm on the Calf		L: R:
7. Using Your Forearm on Hamstrings		L: R:
8. Squeezing the Palm		L: R:
9. Fisting Biceps		L: R:

Position	Time taken	Comments
Supine (continued)		
10. Using Your Forearm on Triceps		L: R:
11. Fisting Pectorals		L: R:
12. Using a Tool on Trapezius		L: R:
13. Applying Digital Pressure to Cervical Muscles		L: R:
14. Applying Digital Pressure to the Occipital Region		L: R:
Prone		
1. Using Your Forearm on the Calf		L: R:
2. Using Your Forearm to Apply Soft Tissue Release		L: R:
3. Using Your Elbow on the Calf		L: R:
4. Calf Squeeze		L: R:
5. Fisting Tibialis Anterior		L: R:
6. Using Your Forearms on Hamstrings		L: R:
7. Using Your Elbows on Hamstrings		L: R:
8. Accessing Piriformis		L: R:
9. Using Your Forearm on Wrist Extensors		L: R:
10. Working the Posterior Shoulder		L: R:
11. Tractioning the Glenohumeral Joint		L: R:
12. Transverse Sretching to Erector Spinae		L: R:
13. Pulling Through Trapezius		L: R:
14. Using Your Forearm on Trapezius		L: R:
15. Accessing Supraspinatus		L: R:
16. Applying Digital Pressure to the Neck Muscles		L: R:

From J. Johnson, 2011, *Deep tissue massage* (Champaign, IL: Human Kinetics).

THREE-QUARTER LYING

This routine includes 12 steps: 6 for the upper body and 6 for the lower body. The 6 upper body steps start at the neck and work to the waist. For the 6 lower body steps, you will start at the ankle and work to the gluteals. If you spend 5 minutes practicing all 12 steps, the routine will take an entire hour. However, this means treating just one side of the body, and it is really helpful to practice applying these techniques to both the left and right sides. What feels comfortable for you to apply to one side of the body using your right arm, for example, might feel awkward (at first) when you need to apply the same technique to the other side of the body using your left arm. It is thus a good idea to spend just a few minutes practicing each technique, then to ask the client to turn over and practice the same techniques on the other side of the body. You might find that to apply these 12 steps alone, to both sides of the body, takes 60 minutes. It is useful to make a note of what time it is before starting these techniques.

1. Using Your Forearm on Upper Trapezius

Start by locating the fleshiest part of your client's upper trapezius muscle and applying compression to it. Rock your forearm over the muscle, getting feedback from the client to identify where pressure feels best.

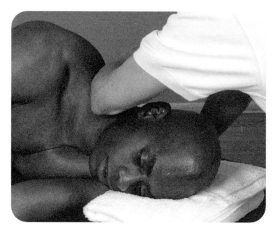

> **Q:** How are you supporting your own back while you apply this stroke? Are you resting one hand on the table? Are you squatting or kneeling?

> **Q:** Does it matter where you stand, squat or kneel in relation to the client?

Next, apply oil to the upper trapezius and shoulder, using your usual massage techniques but with the client in this very different treatment position. As you spread the oil, palpate for the cervical vertebrae plus the spine of the scapulae and the acromion of the scapulae. These are the bony points you are going to avoid applying too much pressure to. When you are ready, start to effleurage using your forearm.

> **Q:** Which movement feels better, sweeping your stroke from the head to the scapulae, or dragging towards you from the scapula to the head?

2. Using Your Elbow on Levator Scapulae

Palpate for the superior angle of the scapulae where the levator scapulae inserts. Place a facecloth or small towel over this area and then gently apply pressure using your elbow. (In the photo, we have removed the facecloth so you can identify the spot to which you apply pressure.)

Q: What happens when you change the angle of your elbow?

Remove the facecloth and soothe the area with massage.

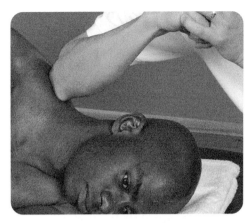

3. Stretching Latissimus Dorsi

You will have some oil on your hands and the shoulder area. Practice this lat stretch first without adding extra oil to the trunk (as shown in the photo), then by adding oil, and finally by placing the facecloth over the area and pressing through it.

Q: Which proves the best way for you to stretch this area—with oil or through a cloth?

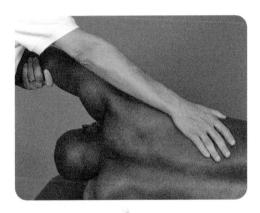

4. Treating the Posterior Shoulder

Thoroughly warm the area with massage, and then practice gently applying pressure through a cloth or towel using your elbow. (In the photo, we have removed the face-cloth so you can identify the spot to which you apply pressure.)

Q: What happens when you passively move the client's arm as you do this?

Remove the towel and soothe the area with massage.

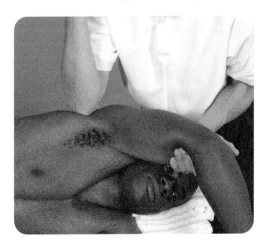

5. Using Your Forearm on Quadratus Lumborum

Work all the way down the thorax to the waist. Once you have applied the oil to this area, practice massaging with your forearms, using one arm to sweep down to the iliac crest (as shown in the photo), or using both arms in a scissor-like action.

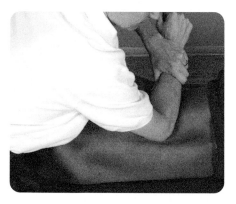

> **Q:** Where do you need to stand to massage this area using your forearms?
>
> **Q:** Do you need to stand with a wider stance to do this?

6. Using Your Elbow on Quadratus Lumborum

When you are sure the area is thoroughly warmed, use the facecloth once again to prevent slipping, and apply pressure to the quadratus lumborum. Be sure to thoroughly soothe the area following pressure. (In the photo, we have removed the facecloth.)

   If necessary, cover the client's upper body now that you have practiced the techniques here and are moving to the lower body.

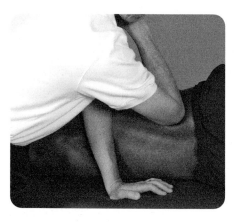

> **Q:** How long did you spend practicing these techniques on the upper body?

Now turn your attention to the client's lower body.

7. Treating the Achilles

Sitting on the edge of the couch, gently take the client's ankle and explore the Achilles tendon. Notice how you can palpate this tendon and possibly work along it and up into the calf in this position.

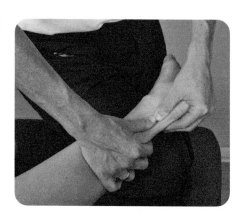

> **Q:** Could you also massage the foot in this position? How about part of the calf?

8. Fisting the Medial Calf

Standing at the foot of the treatment couch, practice slowly fisting up the medial aspect of this muscle, gently compressing it against the couch. Note that by working on the medial side you avoid compression of tissues against the fibula.

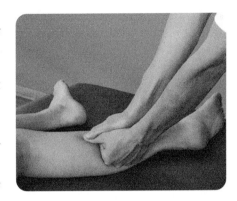

> **Q:** When fisting, does it work better when you cup your right fist or when you cup your left fist?

> **Q:** Are you able to work all the way up the medial calf this way?

Effleurage the area.

9. Using Your Elbow on the Medial Calf

Using oil slowly and carefully, glide your elbow up the medial calf. If needed, use one hand as a guide, similar to the technique shown on page 137.

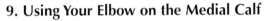

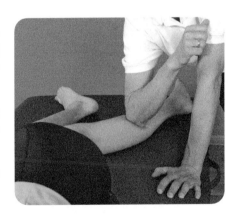

> **Q:** What happens to your posture when you try to apply this technique? What can you do about it?

Soothe the area and glide over the knee to the thigh. Effleurage the inner thigh.

10. Using Your Forearms on Adductors

Now practice effleuraging the inner thigh using your forearm, compressing the muscle against the couch. Remember to avoid pressing too deeply on the medial epicondyle of the femur.

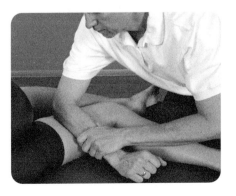

> **Q:** How do you need to stand to effleurage using your forearm?

> **Q:** Can you return to the ankle and find a way to effleurage from the ankle to the calf to the inner thigh, linking together the whole of this lower limb? Do you have to move around the therapy couch to do this?

If necessary, cover the lower limb that you have been massaging (the one resting against the couch) because you are going to move to the uppermost thigh now.

11. Using Your Forearm on the ITB

Massage the lateral thigh using your regular massage strokes, and then use your forearm. This time you need to be careful not to press too deeply into the lateral epicondyle of the femur, close to the knee.

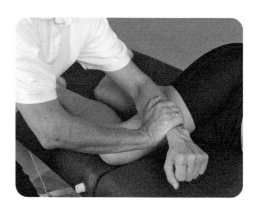

> **Q:** Using which forearm works best for you—your left or your right?
>
> **Q:** What happens when you reinforce your forearm with your other hand?
>
> **Q:** Do you need to stand in a lunge position to apply this technique?

12. Using Your Forearm on Gluteals

You can either massage the gluteals and then place a towel over the area, or simply work through a towel and practice compressing the gluteal muscles using your forearm.

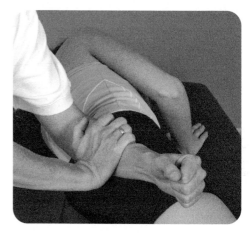

> **Q:** Are you able to identify any area that feels particularly tender for the client? Or any area that they report as feeling good to have compressed in this manner?
>
> **Q:** How long did you spend practicing these techniques on this side of the lower body?

Now help your client turn over, and then return to step 1 to practice the same techniques on their opposite side.

SUPINE

There are 14 steps in this routine: 7 for the lower body and 7 for the upper body.

1. Applying Your Elbow to Tibialis Anterior

After massaging the front of the leg, have a go at stripping the tibialis anterior muscle using your elbow, remembering to go slowly and to guide your elbow using the web of your other hand if necessary.

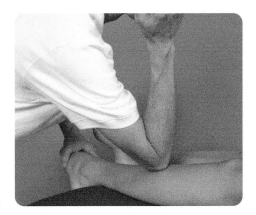

> **Q:** Does it make a difference if your client moves the ankle as you perform this technique?
>
> **Q:** How easy is it to stay on the tibialis anterior muscle?
>
> **Q:** On which part of the muscle does the client report feeling the technique most?

Soothe the area following stripping and link the leg to the thigh with effleurage.

2. Using Your Forearm on the Quadriceps

Warm the quadriceps using your regular strokes of effleurage and petrissage and then practice using your forearms to massage this muscle group.

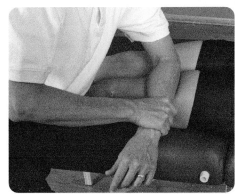

> **Q:** Which forearm do you prefer using? Can you use either?

3. Using Your Forearm on the ITB

Flex the client's knee and, supporting it with one hand, use your forearm to compress and effleurage the iliotibial band and lateral thigh.

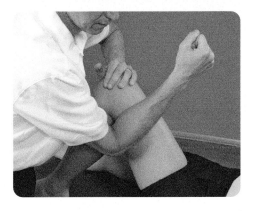

4. Using Your Forearm on the Adductors

Gently abduct the client's hip, allowing the thigh to rest on your knee or supported with bolsters. Taking care not to press too deeply to the medial epicondyle of the femur, practice using your forearm to slowly effleurage the adductors as far as feels appropriate for your client.

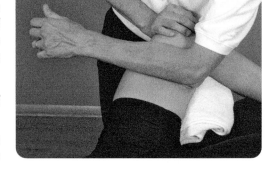

> **Q:** Can you effleurage using either of your forearms?
>
> **Q:** How does your own back feel in this position? Is there anything you can do to safeguard your back?

Q: Which technique does your client prefer? This one or the massage to the adductors technique you performed in the three-quarter-lying position?

Q: In which of these positions do you prefer to treat this muscle group?

5. Calf Squeeze

With the client's knee still flexed, sit on the couch *and* on the client's foot, and gently squeeze the calf muscle. For clients with hairy legs you will need to apply more oil to this area, which you have not yet worked.

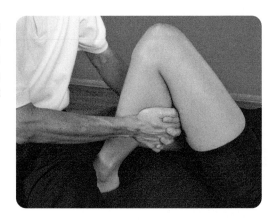

6. Using Your Forearm on the Calf

Practice compressing and effleuraging the calf from ankle to knee, using first one forearm and then the other, changing hands to support the knee as necessary.

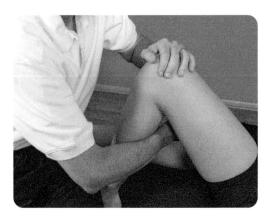

7. Using Your Forearm on Hamstrings

Still sitting on the couch, lift the client's leg and practice using your forearms to massage the hamstrings, working from the knee to the hip.

Q: How does the client feel having the leg elevated in this way?

You can finish this limb by massaging the whole of the front of the leg and thigh, linking ankle to tibialis anterior to quadriceps. It is important to practice delivering the techniques to both sides of the client, so cover this leg and turn to the other side. Once you have finished both lower limbs, turn your attention to the client's upper body.

Q: How long did you spend practicing these techniques to the lower limbs?

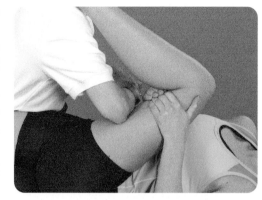

8. Squeezing the Palm

Practice squeezing the palm, ensuring to compress and stretch the thenar and hypothenar eminences.

Q: How do you feel sitting on the side of the couch rather than standing to perform this technique?

Effleurage the whole of the upper limb.

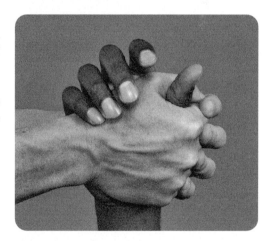

9. Fisting Biceps

Supporting the client's limb, as shown, practice slowly fisting the biceps. Link the hand to the forearm to the arm, taking care not to press into the cubital fossa on the anterior elbow.

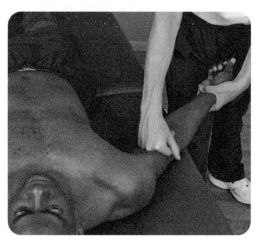

10. Using Your Forearm on Triceps

Find a comfortable position in which to massage the triceps, carefully taking the client's upper limb above the head as shown in the photo. Apply oil, and then practice using your forearm to effleurage. Return the client's arm to the couch, and then once again link the hand to the forearm to the arm.

> **Q:** Which forearm do you prefer to use in this position?

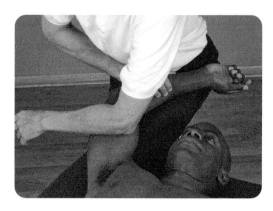

11. Fisting Pectorals

Apply a little oil to the pectoral area; then practice gently fisting the pectorals. The client's arm will be slippery with oil, so you might find it useful to grip gently, using a small towel. (We have omitted the towel in the photo.)

When you have finished, practice steps 8, 9, 10 and 11 to the client's other upper limb.

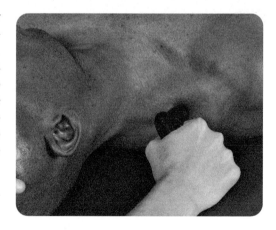

12. Using a Tool on Trapezius

Now that you have massaged both upper limbs, effleurage the neck using whichever techniques you feel appropriate. When you are comfortable that the tissues are warmed and the client is starting to relax, place a small facecloth over the area and gently apply a massage tool to the upper fibers of trapezius. Be sure to soothe the area. (We have omitted the facecloth in the photo.)

> **Q:** How do you need to position yourself to do this? Are you kneeling?

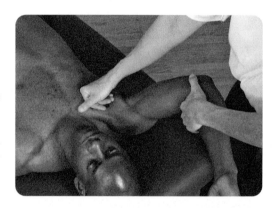

13. Applying Digital Pressure to Cervical Muscles

Gently work into the client's lateral neck, ensuring to avoid deep pressure to the transverse processes of the vertebrae. If you have not done this before, use this session to help you palpate the lateral neck, getting feedback from your client to learn in which parts pressure feels best.

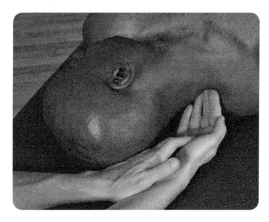

Q: What happens if you kneel down to treat the neck in this way?

Practice steps 12 and 13 on the client's other side.

14. Applying Digital Pressure to the Occipital Region

Finally, use both hands to practice palpating the posterior aspect of your client's neck, gently pulling through the tissues and pressing into the fleshy areas, avoiding the spinous processes of the cervical vertebrae. Allow the weight of the client's head to rest on your fingers. Finish with gentle effleurage.

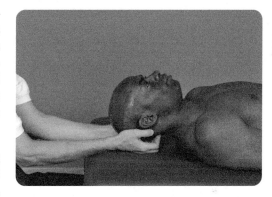

Q: How long did you spend practicing the upper body techniques in supine?

Q: Altogether, how long did it take you to practice these 14 steps on both sides of the body?

PRONE

There are 16 steps in this routine: 8 for the lower limb, 3 for the upper limb and 5 for the trunk.

1. Using Your Forearm on the Calf

Having warmed the muscles using effleurage and petrissage, practice effleurage using your forearm.

Q: Are you able to use either forearm to do this?

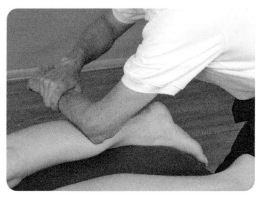

2. Using Your Forearm to Apply Soft Tissue Release

Flexing the client's knee, practice fore-arm effleurage with both active and passive dorsiflexion of the ankle.

> **Q:** How does this feel for the client in comparison to the first step—lighter, deeper or no different?

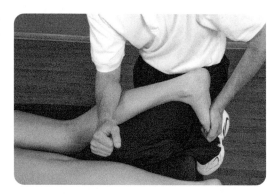

3. Using Your Elbow on the Calf

Once the muscles are fully warmed, use the web of one hand to guide the elbow of your other arm as you practice stripping the calf. Do not press into the popliteal space.

> **Q:** How do you have to stand to safely guard your own posture as you do this?

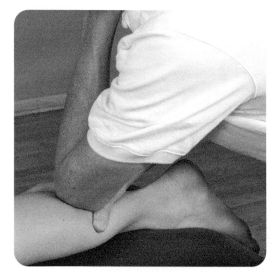

4. Calf Squeeze

Sitting on the couch, soothe and squeeze the calf.

> **Q:** Do you need to add oil to do this?

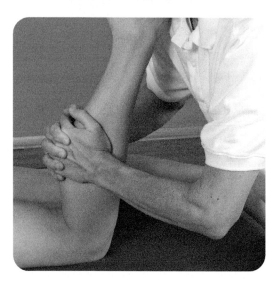

5. Fisting Tibialis Anterior

With the leg in this same position, apply oil and gently fist the tibialis anterior. Return the leg to the couch.

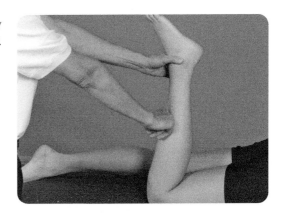

6. Using Your Forearms on Hamstrings

Return to the ankle and link the ankle to the calf to the thigh using effleurage. Then practice using your forearms to effleurage the hamstrings.

> **Q:** How do you have to stand to perform this technique without hurting your own back?

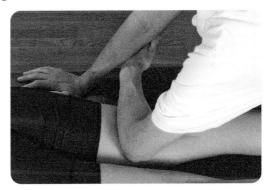

7. Using Your Elbows on Hamstrings

Practice using your elbows on the hamstrings, as shown. When first learning this technique it can be helpful to use the web of your other hand as a guide to prevent you from slipping.

Soothe the hamstrings, and then again link the whole of the lower limb together, effleuraging from the ankle to the calf to the thigh.

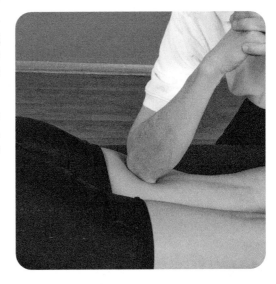

8. Accessing Piriformis

Either massage the buttocks and then apply compression through a towel, or work straight through a towel, remembering to start with minimal pressure. (We have not used a towel in the photo se you can see the proper positioning.)

When finished, soothe the area, cover this limb and practice all techniques on the client's opposite limb.

Q: How long did you spend practicing the techniques on the lower limbs in prone?

When finished, cover both lower limbs and start the next steps, which are for the upper limb.

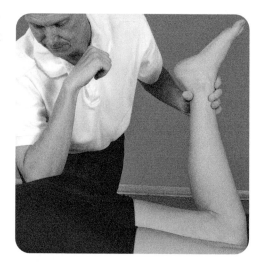

9. Using Your Forearm on Wrist Extensors

With the client's arm positioned as shown, gently effleurage before using your forearm to treat this area.

Q: Does it make a difference if the client moves the wrist as you apply this stroke?

Using your hands, massage into the back of the shoulder.

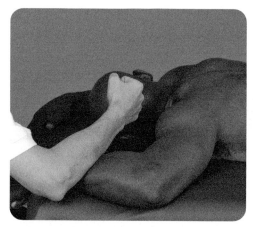

10. Working the Posterior Shoulder

Passively move your client's arm into abduction; then gently apply pressure.

Q: Do you need to kneel to apply this technique? Or stand with a wide stance?

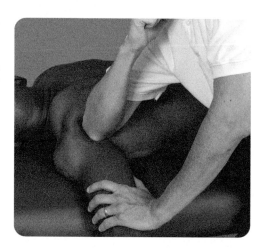

11. Tractioning the Glenohumeral Joint

Holding the client's arm through a towel (if that helps your grip), gently traction the joint.

Practice steps 9, 10 and 11 on the client's other arm.

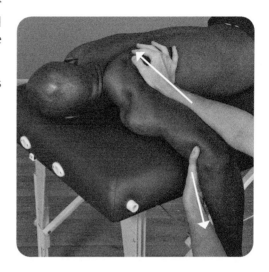

12. Transverse Stretching to Erector Spinae

Apply oil to the back as you normally would. Then place a towel over the client and stretch the erector spinae by pressing transversely across the muscles through the towel. Remove the towel and soothe the area. (We show the technique without the towel to demonstrate the hand position.)

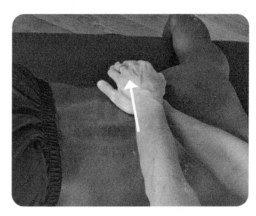

13. Pulling Through Trapezius

Warm the trapezius using your regular strokes; then reinforce your hands and pull through this muscle, leaning back for maximum leverage.

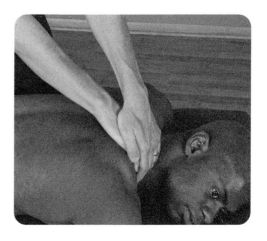

14. Using Your Forearm on Trapezius

Now try something different. Place a small towel or bolster beneath the client's arm and use your forearm to gently glide around the medial border of the scapula. For comparison, try this with and without the supportive towel.

> **Q:** Which method does the client prefer—with or without the towel?
>
> **Q:** Which do you prefer?

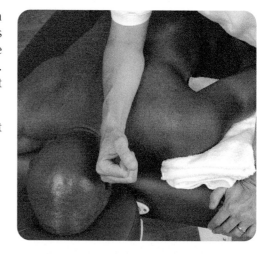

15. Accessing Supraspinatus

Place a facecloth over the upper trapezius. Then gently press into the tissues of this muscle and into supraspinatus, using a tool. Soothe the area following compression. (We have removed the towel so you can see the position of the massage tool.)

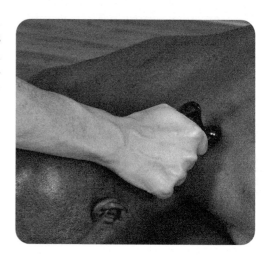

16. Applying Digital Pressure to the Neck Muscles

Finally, practice palpating the posterior neck. Which part of the neck is fleshiest? To which part can you apply slightly deeper pressure than you have been doing?

Now practice steps 12 through 16 on the other side of the body. When finished, link everything together by effleuraging the back and neck.

> **Q:** How long did you spend practicing techniques to the upper body in prone?

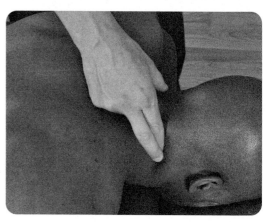

Case Studies

Deep tissue massage may be used to treat a wide range of clients with varying conditions. Presented here are overviews of the way deep tissue massage was used to treat three clients with far-different conditions and using different treatment positions. One client was a female bodybuilder, for whom deep tissue massage later became contraindicated. Another client was a serious runner with a tight iliotibial band that possibly contributed to her knee pain. A third client was a young man who had suffered a fractured wrist while playing tennis. Together these studies illustrate the adaptability of the techniques, highlight certain contraindications and, we hope, inspire you to consider the use of deep tissue massage for the treatment of some of your own clients. A medical history was taken for all clients; there were no initial contraindications to treatment.

Client A: Female Bodybuilder

This client was a 30-year-old female bodybuilder and personal trainer, remarkably with no history of injury. Her request was for a regular series of deep tissue massage treatments, once per week for her back and the back of her lower limbs only. Having had many massage treatments in the past, from many different therapists, she had developed preferences for different muscle groups and requested to have certain parts excluded for the treatment: her gluteals, upper limbs, front of lower limbs and abdomen. By excluding these she felt that the one-hour deep tissue treatment could be better used to address her low back and hamstrings, which she felt were always stiff, and her upper back, which felt okay but which she said other therapists never treated deeply enough for her satisfaction. She went on to explain that it was the sensation of deep tissue massage that she particularly wanted to feel in this region of her upper trapezius and rhomboids. She stated that she liked the sensation of pain here, that when she felt some pain she knew the treatment was working because it felt 'deep enough'.

This was a client with a clear understanding of anatomy and physiology who equated the effectiveness of her treatment with the experience of pain. She had a definite idea of what she wanted from the treatment, and which parts of her body she wanted massaged. At first, Client A appeared to be a client who believed she had to suffer some pain in order to achieve her desired treatment outcome. Further questioning revealed that when she described the 'pain' of deep tissue massage, it was not in terms of something she felt she had to tolerate but more of a pleasurable sensation.

A treatment plan was negotiated. The first session would be used as an assessment for both the client and therapist to identify exactly how much pressure and what types of techniques the client found most pleasurable. We also used this first session to gauge how the client felt remaining in a prone position for an hour. Many clients would feel uncomfortable lying face down for this length of time, and might also experience low back ache caused by the lordotic position of the lumbar spine. The client agreed to place a small pillow beneath her abdomen to reduce the lumbar lordosis.

Following the first session, both Client A and I had a good understanding of what was expected from the treatment. She continued to receive weekly treatments of an almost identical nature, and agreed to having her quadriceps included in the session. However, after almost a year of successful treatment, the client one day arrived with quite severe low back pain of sudden onset for which she had sought medical advice. Despite wanting the same treatment as usual, she agreed to postpone treatment until she had received a diagnosis for her back pain. This was later revealed to be a serious condition—a result of overloading the vertebrae with heavy weights, totally contraindicated for massage of the low back and also contraindicated for resting in a prone position.

The client did not wish to receive any other form of massage to other parts of her body, so a decision was made not to continue providing deep tissue massage for this client. The client was disappointed but eventually acquiesced to my need to adhere to professional guidelines regarding conditions contraindicated to massage.

Client B: Serious Runner

Client B was a female client who regularly took part in marathons and half-marathons. She had been experiencing a niggling pain on the lateral side of her left knee and wanted massage to make it go away. She explained how she used to rub the side of her thigh and that this had helped in the past, but this time it had failed to take her knee pain away. The client was already doing active stretches for the iliotibial band and gluteals which, she felt did 'not really do much'. A series of standard knee tests were performed, all of which were negative. However, the Ober test and palpation revealed a very tight iliotibial band. It was proposed that the tight band could be contributing to the problem perhaps by rubbing on the lateral epicondyle, exactly where she was getting her pain. I showed her a picture of the band and the tensor fascia latae and gluteus maximus muscles attached to it. I explained that to alleviate tension in the band it would be necessary to treat these muscles, plus the quadriceps.

The client agreed and consented to having her right leg treated also. She had three sessions, each of just 40 minutes (20 minutes on each thigh) including static pressure to the tensor fascia latae muscle and gluteals, over a period of 15 days (approximately one session every 5 days), during which time she agreed to reduce the number of miles she was running. This client was happy to take an active part in her treatment and was not keen on massage for the sake of relaxation. She enjoyed having forearm massage to the lateral thigh in three-quarter lying, in which position she was able to actively flex and extend her knee. I was also able to access the tensor fascia latae and gluteals in this position.

The pain resolved following three sessions of deep tissue massage, and I advised her to return for maintenance treatment once a month. I also showed her how to apply static pressure to the tensor fascia latae muscle herself.

Client C: Wrist Injury

Client C was a male who had fractured his left forearm when he fell playing tennis. He had been in a cast for six weeks. When the cast was removed, he attended two sessions of physical therapy and admitted to 'not really doing the exercises'. His wrist was pain free but stiff, and he wanted to get back to playing tennis. Fortunately, the left hand was not his dominant hand. Range-of-movement tests revealed that he had lost range in all movements of the wrist: flexion, extension, radial and ulnar deviation. He had full finger flexion but reduced extension in the metacarpophalangeal joints of all fingers.

The client agreed to and received deep tissue massage to his upper limb, focusing on the forearm flexors and extensors. Range of motion at the wrist and metacarpophalangeal joints was measured before and after each treatment, which was administered weekly for six weeks. After six weeks, range of movement was significantly improved, and he was able to make a complete return to tennis.

Closing Remarks

Now that you have practiced the techniques in the form of routines and read the case studies, you should have an abundance of ideas for incorporating deep tissue massage techniques into your own practice. The world of deep tissue therapy and bodywork is diverse and continually evolving. The ideas put forward in this book have served me well and I hope will be of value to readers. As a practicing therapist myself, I welcome comments, questions and suggestions from other therapists. Please feel free to get in touch with me if you would like to share your experiences of the use of deep tissue massage.

Answers to Quick Questions

Chapter 1

1. The two main techniques for delivering deep tissue massage covered in this book are *compression* and *stretch*.

2. To increase the sensation of pressure for a client wanting deep tissue massage you could do any of the following:
   - Apply more pressure.
   - Keep the pressure the same, but reduce the surface area to which you are applying it.
   - Apply more pressure *and* reduce the surface area to which you are applying it.
   - Have the client contract the muscle that works opposite to the one you are treating.
   - Give the impression of deep pressure without physically pressing into tissues more deeply by adding a stretching component.

3. Sports massage and deep tissue massage are not the same. Deep tissue massage techniques are one set of techniques used by sports massage therapists but may also be used by other therapists wanting to apply deeper massage.

4. The answer to this question depends on you, the reader!

5. Three conditions that make some deep tissue massage techniques suitable for inclusion in a chair massage routine even though they can be sedative are the following:
   - Seated chair massage routines tend to be shorter in duration than Swedish massage routines.
   - The intention of the therapist providing chair massage is not usually deep relaxation.
   - Chair massage routines frequently end with a few minutes of upbeat tapotement to help acclimatize the client back to the work environment.

Chapter 2

1. Three questions you might ask concerning the no-pain-no-gain approach are these:
   - Is it ethical?
   - Is it legal?
   - Does it *really* work better than deep tissue techniques applied without pain?

2. A treatment goal for the use of deep tissue massage might be . . .
   - to alleviate cramp,
   - to facilitate the treatment of trigger spots,
   - to improve range in a joint,
   - to facilitate deep relaxation,
   - to address tension in a particular muscle group,
   - to overcome musculoskeletal imbalance, or
   - to help improve posture.

3. Positive emotional states from which to choose an intention prior to massage could be any of the following:
   Calm
   Caring
   Compassionate
   Confident
   Conscientious
   Creative
   Effective
   Energized
   Grounded
   Optimistic
   Positive
   Sensitive

4. One simple thing you can do with your treatment couch to facilitate deep tissue massage is to lower it by 2 inches (5 cm).

5. Some possible side effects of deep tissue massage are
   - dizziness and disorientation,
   - bruising and
   - feelings in muscles similar to delayed onset muscle soreness (DOMS).

Chapter 3

1. When using forearm techniques, the client will experience an increase in pressure if you clench the fist of the forearm you are using.

2. One of the difficulties inherent to the application of fisting techniques is for therapists to maintain their wrists in neutral while also keeping their elbows straight.

3. In addition to leaning more heavily onto the client, simply flexing the elbow by a few degrees will hugely increase the pressure felt by the client.

4. To prevent the elbow from slipping when using the elbow to apply a stripping technique, it is necessary to reinforce the elbow using the web of the other hand.

5. Of all of the techniques described here, using forearms are best for the application of broad, relatively diffuse compression, while the use of massage tools (or an elbow) works better for treating a small, specific spot.

Chapter 4

1. When using dry stretching, the sensation of deep pressure can be enhanced by adding a small amount of oil to the area being treated, and then applying the stretch through a facecloth or small towel.

2. Tractioning is not appropriate for the following clients: clients who are hypermobile or who have been diagnosed with having a hypermobile syndrome; clients who have suffered dislocated joints or who have joint instability; clients with known inflammatory joint conditions; clients with ankylosing spondylitis or fused joints; clients with fragile skin.

3. The advantage of asking the client to actively move a joint during a stretch with oil is that this helps decrease muscle tone in the muscle being stretched.

4. When treating the wrist extensors, you position the client with the wrist off the end of the treatment couch so you can move the joint into flexion.

5. It is difficult to apply passive joint movement when the therapist has limited leverage with which to apply compressive massage strokes.

Chapter 5

1. When using your elbow to treat the quadratus lumborum muscle with your client in the three-quarter-lying position, it is best to avoid deep pressure to the ribs and kidney area.

2. When treating the upper fibers of trapezius with a client in supine, use a massage tool to compress tissues for up to 30 seconds.

3. When treating the diaphragm, pressure is applied as the client exhales.

4. To increase grip when treating the erector spinae muscles transversely with a client in the prone position, simply apply a little oil to the skin and press through a facecloth or small towel.

5. When treating rhomboids and upper trapezius muscles of a client in prone position, placing a towel or bolster beneath the shoulder passively shortens the upper fibers of the trapezius and sometimes the rhomboids, allowing easier access to these muscles.

Chapter 6

1. When treating the adductors in three-quarter-lying position, it is possible to also access the hamstrings.

2. To introduce an element of stretch when treating hamstrings in supine using the forearm or elbow, ask the client to straighten his or her knee as you perform the stroke.

3. To locate the tensor fascia latae muscle in supine, ask the client to take his or her leg off the couch and internally rotate the hip.

4. When squeezing the calf with the client prone, it is important to work from the ankle to the knee to aid venous and lymphatic drainage.

5. When treating hamstrings in prone with an elbow, end the massage stroke at the ischium, if possible.

Chapter 7

1. In an attempt to access the subscapularis muscle in the three-quarter-lying position it is necessary to press through the middle fibers of the trapezius and the rhomboid muscles as well as their surrounding fascia.

2. When treating the triceps in supine using either the forearm or fist, it is best to avoid localized deep pressure to the armpit itself.

3. Two techniques that could be used to treat the hand of a client in supine are fisting and squeezing.

4. To locate the supraspinatus muscle with the client in the prone position, find the V shape formed by the junction of the spine of the scapula with the acromion process. Supraspinatus lies in the supraspinous fossa deep to the upper fibers of the trapezius.

5. If a client tenses during the application of pressure to the infraspinatus muscle in prone, stop the procedure, soothe the area and start again.

PRONE

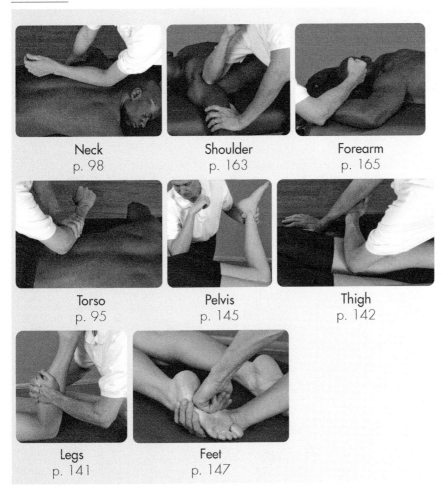

Neck
p. 98

Shoulder
p. 163

Forearm
p. 165

Torso
p. 95

Pelvis
p. 145

Thigh
p. 142

Legs
p. 141

Feet
p. 147

SITTING

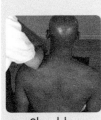

Shoulder
p. 101

SUPINE

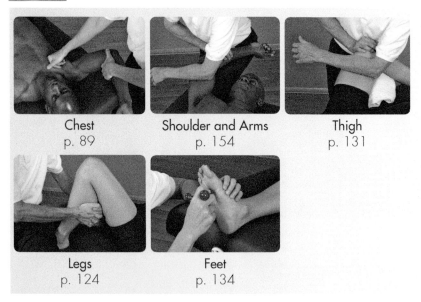

Chest
p. 89

Shoulder and Arms
p. 154

Thigh
p. 131

Legs
p. 124

Feet
p. 134

THREE-QUARTER LYING

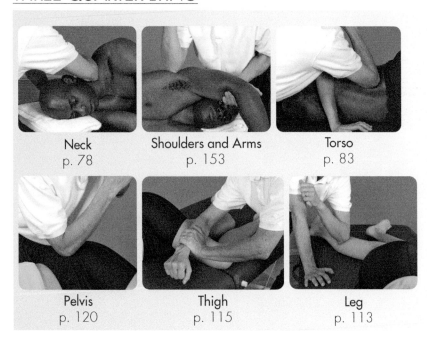

Neck
p. 78

Shoulders and Arms
p. 153

Torso
p. 83

Pelvis
p. 120

Thigh
p. 115

Leg
p. 113

About the Author

Jane Johnson, MSc, is director of the London Massage Company in London, England. As a chartered physiotherapist and sports massage therapist, she has been using and teaching deep tissue massage (DTM) for many years and has a thorough grounding in anatomy, which she uses to explain DTM in straightforward terms. She has worked with numerous client groups, including athletes, recreational exercisers, office workers and older adults. This experience has enabled her to adapt DTM for various types of clients and provide tips for readers. Johnson has taught advanced massage skills for many years and has worked as a fitness instructor, massage therapist and physiotherapist. She frequently presents at conferences and exhibitions for therapists.

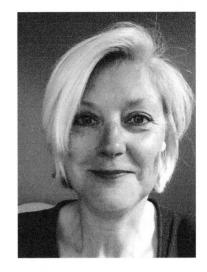

Johnson is a full member of the Chartered Society of Physiotherapists and is registered with the Health Professions Council. She is a consultant and examiner in sports massage for the Association of Physical and Natural Therapists and is a member of the Institute of Anatomical Sciences. In her leisure time, she enjoys writing articles and newsletters for therapists, taking her dog for long walks and visiting museums and exhibitions relating to human sciences.

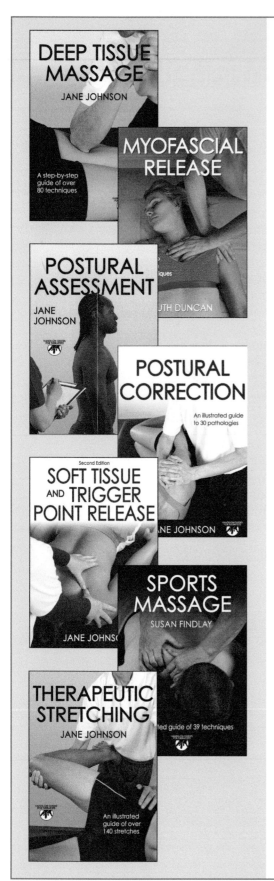

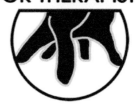
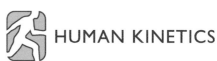